Multiple Sclerosis

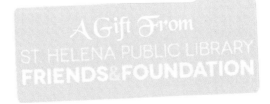

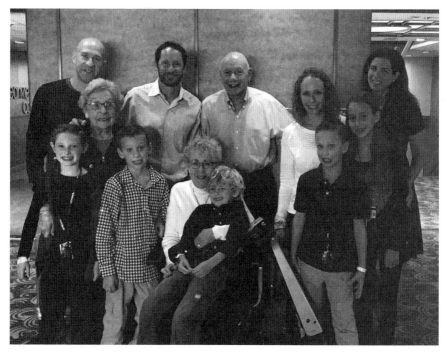

The author and her family on an Alaskan cruise in August 2016.

Multiple Sclerosis

Tips and Strategies for Making Life Easier

Third Edition

Shelley Peterman Schwarz

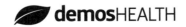 **demos**HEALTH

Visit our website at www.demoshealth.com

ISBN: 9780826156334
eISBN: 9780826156341

Acquisitions Editor: Beth Barry
Compositor: diacriTech

Library of Congress Cataloging-in-Publication Data
Names: Schwarz, Shelley Peterman, author.
Title: Multiple sclerosis : tips and strategies for making life easier /
    Shelley Peterman Schwarz.
Description: Third edition. | New York : Demos Health, [2017] | Includes
    bibliographical references and index.
Identifiers: LCCN 2017011331 | ISBN 9780826156334 | ISBN 9780826156341 (e-ISBN)
Subjects: LCSH: Multiple sclerosis--Popular works.
Classification: LCC RC377 .S26 2017 | DDC 616.8/34--dc23 LC record available at
https://lccn.loc.gov/2017011331

Printed in the United States of America by McNaughton & Gunn.
17 18 19 20 21 / 5 4 3 2 1

Contents

A Word From the Author

The world and I have both changed a lot in the 10 years since I wrote the second edition of *Multiple Sclerosis: 300 Tips for Making Life Easier*. Now 10 years older and, I hope, a little wiser, I felt that this NEW book had to go beyond the tips and strategies of the original book. I wanted this book to include more personal, real-life stories and experiences from my 38 years of living with multiple sclerosis (MS).

I also wanted to answer the following important questions (and so many more):

- How do you stay positive and keep motivated when life is no longer under your control and the "rules of the game" keep changing?
- What do you do when family and friends don't understand what you're going through?
- How do you stay involved when you're no longer able to do what you once did?
- How do you bounce back when MS knocks you down, over and over again?
- How do you remain a responsible parent when you don't have any energy or stamina?

When I started my MS journey in 1979, I didn't know that I would become severely disabled. (Remember, this was before any of the medications to treat MS were developed. And, because of my primary progressive MS diagnosis, I never qualified for the treatments that were developed.)

In the beginning, I lost physical abilities every day. I tried to keep up and find new ways of doing things. I've always been a positive person and a lifelong problem solver, but the daily struggles were a real test to my ingenuity. I had to find ways of consolidating, streamlining, and rearranging the way I did simple everyday tasks. Each time I have faced a problem that MS imposed, such as dressing myself independently, I took it as a personal challenge.

I began developing my own tips, techniques, and time-savers and soon realized that everyone has his or her own ideas for making life easier. I became a keen observer of how other people did things. Even today I look at obstacles and inabilities as problems waiting for a solution. After years of all sorts of personal and professional challenges, I have discovered that I can be quite creative and resourceful. There are not many things I "can't" do, and I hope you will find this, too.

What I also learned was that my attitude and outlook were even more important to my well-being than all the tips and time-savers. I had to adapt and develop new skills and strategies to handle everyday situations that made me feel sad, frustrated, lonely, and that diminished my self-worth.

When you have MS, you never forget that you are living with a chronic, progressively disabling disease. Yet, despite all the challenges, I'm happier now than I have ever been before, and I live a remarkably unlimited life. I hope the ideas and information in the book encourage and inspire you to make yourself a priority and do the things you need to do to be happy and enjoy life.

In the not-too-distant future, medical science will find a cure for MS and we owe it to ourselves to be in the best mental and physical shape possible when that day comes.

I leave you with the words I live by . . .

When you live with love and gratitude in your heart, you transform yourself and the people around you!

I wish you the best on your journey,

Shelley Peterman Schwarz

Acknowledgments

Judy Ross, thank you for being my mentor, sounding board, cheerleader, and dear friend.

Deborah Proctor, thank you for working on this project with me. Your help was invaluable.

David Schwarz, there are no words to adequately thank you for giving me the freedom to live my life to the fullest. YOU are a remarkable man!

To all my wonderful friends and neighbors: Please know that I couldn't do what I do without you, and you have my deepest, heartfelt thanks.

Multiple Sclerosis

CHAPTER 1

Basic Principles for Living With MS

Being diagnosed with MS forced me to simplify my life. I was 32 years old, and it was clear that life as I knew it had changed forever. As much as I wanted to deny it, I could not physically, mentally, or emotionally keep up the break-neck pace I demanded of myself. Over the years, I realized there were several basic concepts for conserving time and energy. Using these techniques and strategies, you will be more organized, able to work smarter, and most important, be more independent than you otherwise would have been.

1. Keep balance in your life. Prioritize, eliminate, consolidate, and streamline activities in all aspects of your life.

2. Plan ahead. Be sensible about how you spend your time and energy. Do those things that are most important to you and to your family. Try to eliminate unnecessary or difficult tasks.

3. Alternate periods of activity with periods of rest. Pace your activities. Try to break an activity down into a series of smaller tasks. Rest before you become exhausted and, if need be, enlist the help of others.

4. Eat a healthy diet. Do not skip meals. Carry trail mix, nuts, and/or fresh fruit with you. Eat a healthy snack, and avoid the temptation to grab a candy bar with hollow calories and little nutritional value.

5. Arrange and organize your home for your convenience. Sometimes, this means putting furniture in strategic locations to help you walk from room to room or placing a chair halfway down a long hallway so that you can stop to rest. Sometimes, it means purchasing duplicate cleaning supplies for both upstairs and downstairs rooms.

6. Accept the fact that you need help from time to time. We all do, whether we have MS or not. Don't look at it as giving in. Instead, look at it as making an intelligent decision that will make your life easier and safer.

7. Smart-home technology makes it possible to adjust the heat, lights, ceiling fans, sound, and even open or lock doors from the comfort of your bed or easy chair. Remote-controlled devices, cordless phones, and cell phones save steps.

8. Computers are good for keeping records, journals, and writing letters—which can even be done hands-free with voice-activated software. Synchronize your computer with your cell phone and tablet to keep track of appointments and your schedule.

9. Apps for your smartphone or tablet can help you communicate from one part of the house to another, indoors or out; monitor the safety of a loved one in another room or from afar; turn your smartphone into a flashlight; let you keep track of the news and weather (even alert you to approaching bad storms); and listen to the radio or watch TV or movies.

10. Keep abreast of changes in technology by visiting your computer store, big-box store, or phone carrier and ask for assistance on which software or apps might work best for you. Make full use of every option and new app that might be helpful to you.

11. An Internet connection can expand your research capabilities and provide opportunities to communicate with others who have MS.

12. Stay safe by keeping in touch. Walkie-talkies, which don't require an Internet connection, and smartphones can help you communicate around the house or while shopping, traveling, at museums, theme parks, art shows, or anywhere you might become separated from others in your group. Walkie-talkies are sold at electronic, discount, or office-supply stores. Turn your cell phone into a walkie-talkie by downloading an app from your mobile phone app store.

13. Use labor-saving devices. Many labor-saving devices are available to make almost any task easier. Automatic can and jar openers, toothpaste twisters, hair dryer holders, and quick-release mops are just a few of the many products that may make everyday tasks easier for you to accomplish.

14. Purchase reachers and keep them where you need them to extend your reach or help you pick up or grasp objects. Reachers come in various lengths, weights, and means of operation. Some have trigger grips, similar to a pistol's, which are operated by squeezing your finger. Others have full-grasp handgrips that allow you to squeeze with all your fingers. Some reachers have magnets at the end for picking up metal objects. Others have rubber grippers or vinyl-covered tips for better holding power. Some reachers fold in half for traveling or storage, and some come with a carrying attachment that clamps the reacher to a walker or wheelchair.

15. Conserve energy whenever and wherever possible. Pushing a grocery cart may give you added stability as you walk. If fatigue is a problem, use a wheelchair or scooter whenever walking distances is required. A growing number of stores, shopping malls, museums, zoos, art galleries, and attractions provide battery-operated scooters or wheelchairs for patrons who tire easily or have trouble walking. Scooters and wheelchairs usually are available on a first-come-first-served basis at the service desk or information booth.

16. Before going out, call ahead to a restaurant, theater, new doctor's office, and so forth, and ask whether the facility is

handicap-accessible. Ask about parking facilities, where the restrooms are located, the most convenient entrance—anything that might create a challenge or is of concern to you.

17. If noisy environments in restaurants, grocery stores, and department stores exhaust you, select quieter places in which to spend your time. Look for places with drapes, low ceilings, and carpeted or vinyl floors that absorb the sound; avoid establishments that have wooden floors, walls of windows, loud background music, multiple TVs, or high unfinished ceilings. As an added safeguard, carry earplugs in your purse or pocket.

CHAPTER 2

The Thriver's Guide

In this life, we don't always understand why things happen the way they do. It's human nature to ask, "Why did I get multiple sclerosis? What did I do to deserve this? Did I do something wrong?" There are no answers to these questions. So, when I was diagnosed with MS the questions I struggled with were, "How was my life to have meaning? What was the purpose? What was I supposed to learn?"

The biggest challenge of my life has been finding peace with my life as a woman with a severe disability, a wife, mother, grandmother, daughter, sister, friend, neighbor, and coworker.

Philosophically, I believe that there were/are important lessons for me to learn in my life and MS provided the school. To this day, I continue to learn about myself, my strength, and how resilient I am. MS has also taught me lessons in compassion, humility, and gratitude.

The following essays share how I have learned to live and "thrive" despite the challenges I've faced. I hope these stories, examples, and real-life experiences provide validation, hope, and encouragement to you and reinforce that you too cannot only survive MS, you can THRIVE!

Accepting the "New You"

Every August, the month of my diagnosis, I "celebrate" the anniversary of my life with MS. "Celebrate" seems like a strange word to use around an illness that at onetime left me with no use of my legs and only limited use of my left hand. Yet, it's true. I do celebrate my life, limitations and all. So how does one come to this level of acceptance? As you might guess, it was not easy and it **did not** happen overnight.

Whether it was a small loss like not being able to cut my own food or a large loss like no longer being able to walk, I was in a constant state of grieving. Frustrated by my lack of control, I was petrified of the future. It wasn't easy to stay positive, and I can tell you I threw many a "pity party" where I was the guest of honor.

Yet, somewhere inside of me a little voice said, "I don't want to be sad and unhappy. It's too painful." It took me a long time to understand that if I wanted to heal the emotional pain of my losses, I was going to have to work on changing the way I dealt with life.

So I began making an effort to participate in activities with family and friends, even if all I could do was sit and watch them bowl, dance, or garden.

I tried to participate in household activities—folding clothes and drying dishes, even if I couldn't do the laundry or cook the meal.

I traded in my leadership role in organizational work for a "supporting cast" position, making phone calls and setting up meetings. I enjoyed the involvement and people were happy to have my help.

I've learned that my self-worth and value are not contingent on my physical condition. Living with MS has taught me that having time for people and relationships is a gift of immense proportion. In my world, that's cause for celebration!

Reassessing What's Important

I used to think that life was about giving to and doing for others. It wasn't until I was "in a wheelchair with one hand tied behind my back" (i.e., severely disabled) that I realized that it's relationships and our ability to connect with those we love and care about that gives our life meaning.

Right before my father passed away, he told me that one of the reasons he fell in love with my mother was because she was such a good listener. Looking back, I now understand that I learned how to be a good listener from my mother.

In fact, my family always teases me because I have an uncanny way of connecting with everyone from good friends to recent acquaintances. Whether it is the air-conditioning repair man, the person who sold me a pair of shoes, or the checker at the grocery store, people share with me intimate details of their life.

I began to wonder why people opened up to me so easily and I came to this simple conclusion: People are so busy running through life that they don't have time to stop and truly listen to each other. Because I can't race through life, I have the time to lend a listening ear.

Perhaps my father had discovered the reason why we have two ears, but only one mouth—we are supposed to listen twice as much as we talk.

Being a good listener is the most important lesson of all and a simple way we can repay, respect, and reward the people who make a difference in our lives.

Telling Family and Friends How They Can Help

We're "lucky"; we have a diagnosis and our illness is one that people have heard of. It validates our complaints and symptoms and adds credibility to our limitations. Our friends and loved ones want to be helpful and lend their support. It's our responsibility to share with people how they can help us.

Many years ago, a girlfriend told me about her husband who had gone into the kitchen to get himself a drink. She mentioned to her husband that she, too, was thirsty. When her husband returned with his drink, but not one for her, she snapped at him for not bringing her a drink.

So often, we expect people to read our minds, when we really have not been clear about what we want. We have to be specific.

I loved it when my parents came to visit from their home 90 miles away. They were willing to help and did so in many ways: like taking care of the children, helping with meal preparation, and doing household tasks. They were wonderful. But . . .

I'd see the anguish in my father's eyes as he fought back tears watching me struggle to do things that once were easy. The steady decline in my physical abilities was painfully obvious and I finally worked up the courage to say the words I needed to say. "Dad, I can't stand to see you cry whenever you look at me. Cry on your way here and on your way home, but, please, don't cry in front of me. This is hard enough without seeing how painful this is for you."

When we express our thoughts and feelings in clear, caring, and loving ways, we strengthen our relationships.

Staying Connected and Involved

"I'll just stay home," was my immediate response when activities were planned. "Really, just go without me. I'll be fine by myself," I reassured my family and friends. But the truth was I was not happy that my world was getting smaller. And I was the person responsible for making it that way.

When I found my world shrinking, I pushed myself to invite good friends over for lunch even though they had to help prepare, serve, and clean it up. At first, I was embarrassed asking my friends to make their lunch and mine, but I learned that they loved being able to help and were happy that I wanted to continue our friendship. Being with good friends was a brief respite from my worries.

More than 30 years ago, I invited a group of women over to play cards. The game was, and still is, always at my house because then I don't have to stress about accessibility issues, the weather, and if I need to lie down, I can, while the game continues. Over the years, we've shared lots of memories and belly laughs. Members of the group take turns bringing refreshments. And the women understand that if I'm having a bad MS day and not up to having the game, someone else hosts the game at their house.

Several years ago, a young immigrant from Armenia came to visit me to practice her English. Now an American citizen, she recently told me, "I can never repay your kindness. As long as I am alive, you will never be alone." Her words touched my heart and brought tears to my eyes. And all I did was invite her to my house to talk!

When I don't feel up to being social with my friends and neighbors, I can connect on my own time by "talking" with folks on the Internet. In addition to using the Internet to connect with others who have chronic illness, I've used the Internet to locate former classmates, people I used to work with, and long-lost relatives. Day or night, I can stay connected to the world beyond me.

It's not fair that we have a chronic illness. However, we owe it to ourselves to reach in and reach out. Our lives will be more fulfilling, more interesting, and we won't get stuck feeling sorry for ourselves and "our lot in life."

Making Compromises

Life is full of compromises. But I wasn't interested. I was angry, stubborn, and I was not going to give in to MS! I was not going to use a #!%#&!# wheelchair! I wasn't going to be one of "those people." Does that sound familiar? Whether it's wearing hearing aids, using oxygen (at home or in public), or an ankle/foot orthotic (AFO) with "dorky-looking" shoes to help (me) with foot drop, it's not easy to accept our limitations no matter how old we are.

I remember when my father-in-law, who was in his 70s and had Parkinson's disease, refused to use a wheelchair when we went to the National Aquarium in Baltimore, Maryland. We were visiting from Wisconsin and wanted to take our 14- and 12-year-old children to see the sites. We knew that if Grandpa wanted to join us, he'd have to use a wheelchair. If he didn't, he would have ended up sitting on a bench in the lobby waiting for us.

At the time, I was 42 and had been using a three-wheeled, battery-operated Amigo® scooter wheelchair (www.myamigo.com) for several years. I remembered how hard it was for me to accept using a wheelchair. In fact, years earlier, we had gone with my in-laws and the children to an amusement park. By the time we walked from the parking lot to the park entrance, I was exhausted. I found a bench and never left it the entire day. The family, at my urging, went on without me. I REFUSED TO USE A WHEELCHAIR! Even though it meant missing out on all the family fun.

I reminded my father-in-law of that day and asked whether he remembered how he felt leaving me on that park bench while he and the children went off to see the sites. He did. And so he (reluctantly) agreed to use the wheelchair. Halfway through the aquarium, my father-in-law gave me a wink and a smile and said, "I could get used to this."

Making compromises is not easy. However, if we don't, we put limits on our lives and miss out on wonderful opportunities and priceless memories.

Asking for Help

Before I started using a wheelchair, I was out with some close friends. To get to our destination, I had to go down some terrace steps. I was unsteady on my feet normally and was terrified that I would fall down the steps (in front of everyone) because there was no railing for me to hang onto. I stood at the top of the stairs paralyzed with fear. Engrossed in conversation, my friends kept walking, until one turned to look to see where I was. In that split second, I made the decision to ask my friend if I could take her arm so I would have the extra support I needed. I made it down safely and looked around. No one was staring at me. No one cared that I needed help. People were "in their own little world." Wow! Was that an "ah ha! moment" for me and a paradigm shift in my thinking.

I've asked for lots of help over the years and have never been turned down, even in the most embarrassing circumstances, like the time I was downtown at one of the state office buildings for a meeting. My friend had dropped me off so I was on my own. As I entered the building, I felt the need to use the ladies room. I started getting panicky because I wasn't with anybody who could help me. As I walked past different offices, I realized that if I didn't want to find myself in a horribly compromised situation, I'd better ask someone to help me.

And that's what I did. I approached a woman behind the desk in one of the offices and told her I needed help and asked whether she would mind helping. At first, she only thought I was looking for a ladies restroom. I explained how I needed a little more help than that. She looked me in the eyes and said, "Of course! What can I do to help you?"

When I was back in my wheelchair, waiting for the elevator to take me up to my meeting, these words echoed in my mind: When you ask for help, someone will always be there to help you.

No, it hasn't been easy! I hate the fact that I need so much help; but when I stop to think about it, asking for help has given me a lot more freedom and, perhaps, people are learning some compassion for others, something our world desperately needs.

Letting Go

Someone once asked me what was the most important lesson I have learned on my MS journey. I knew the answer immediately: learning to **LET GO**. Examples of that surface every day and are constant reminders of its importance.

In the early years of my diagnosis, my hands were becoming weak and stiff, which meant that someone had to spread cream cheese, peanut butter, mustard, and so on, on my bread or crackers. At the time, it seemed like a small, petty problem; but it bothered me because we all have personal preferences, especially when it comes to food. And, even though I asked the person helping me to put on "a thin layer of peanut butter," it didn't turn out that way.

For me, it was the reality of "another loss." Losing abilities and becoming disabled was emotionally painful. Learning to "let go" eased the pain.

I haven't driven a car since 1985, so when relatives, friends, and neighbors drive me in my ramp-equipped van, they choose the route (through town or on the highway), the amount of time we need to get to our destinations given weather or road conditions, and where we should park. I give them the control. I've learned that some drivers know exactly where we're going and don't need any directions, whereas others want me to tell them every turn and lane change, no matter how many times we have gone to the same place. Some worry and need constant reassurance. Some go a little faster than I would if I were driving, whereas others barely keep up. Accepting that others do things differently and letting go has reduced my impatience and frustration.

I've also learned to let go of perfection. So what if some of my drawers are not picture-perfect? I've given myself permission to just toss my underwear, socks, and nightgowns into the drawer. My rationale: Who cares? And it saves time and energy for more important things.

Putting Yourself First

I was a doer. I was always taking care of other people. I rarely thought about my needs or my wants. Who had time? I was too busy.

And then MS put an end to my life as a doer. I had to learn an important new lesson for living, and it was not easy. What was this lesson? You **MUST** take care of yourself by putting your needs first.

I am not suggesting that you be mean, thoughtless, demanding, or selfish. I only encourage you to love yourself enough to "take care of you" and do things that bring love and joy into your life. Most important: Give yourself permission to get rid of "toxic" people in your life. If you cannot eliminate them entirely, reduce your exposure or "dilute their toxicity" by including others when you must be together. People who are negative or pessimistic drain your energy and pull you down.

Having my nails done is one way I take care of myself. I have always wanted nice-looking nails. When my hands lost their strength, my nails started to grow out. Today, my pretty (red) nails put a big smile on my face. Over the years, my girlfriends and I have gone to the local beauty college to get manicures. The cost is nominal and I have met dozens of terrific young men and women.

Putting yourself in positive, uplifting situations and surrounding yourself with good people will help you let go of your anger, frustration, and disappointment over "what might have been." When you make room for smiles and laughter, people want to be around you and include you in their lives.

Talking to Yourself

I start my day with a personal pep talk. Each morning when I look in the bathroom mirror at my bedraggled mop of (naturally) curly hair and baggy/saggy eyes, I could say, "You are one scary lady!" But before I allow my mind to go there, I say in an upbeat voice, "Good morning, Sunshine! Happy (Satur)day! I'm a valuable, worthwhile person and I'm ready to face the world and the challenges that come my way."

Going through my morning routine, I focus on sending positive messages to myself: "That pink turtleneck I'm wearing looks good on me." "The fog and humidity in the air today will make my curls even curlier." "I like these new glasses; they frame my face nicely."

As I put the finishing touches on my hair and makeup, I look at my reflection in the mirror and utter these exact words. "You look great! Shelley, I love you. Now, go and make it a wonderful day!"

My children would be horrified to hear that I talk to myself like that; they'd think I've gone over the edge with my own self-importance. But I'd beg to differ.

I will admit that when I started these morning rituals, I felt foolish, even embarrassed by how ridiculous it sounded. But on the days that I forget, I actually feel less positive and energetic.

Other things I say to myself . . .

When life threatens to overwhelm me, I repeat a mantra. Sometimes that mantra is, "Keep breathing. Keep breathing." Sometimes it's, "Just do one thing." And sometimes it's, "You're gonna be fine."

I also refuse to "should" on myself. Phrases like I *should* write, I *should* call, I *should* send, I *should* go, I *should* make, and so on are no longer in my vocabulary. When you remove the negative "should," you can change the phrase to a more neutral or positive statement.

I pay attention to what my body tells me. If, for example, I'm tired because I didn't sleep well, I'll take a nap. I do not allow myself any negative or judgmental self-talk. I kindly give myself permission to "take care of me." After all, if I don't "take care of me," who will? Slowing down means I get more done. I make fewer mistakes, use less energy, and reduce my stress and tension overall.

We send ourselves messages all the time. Doesn't it make sense to give ourselves loving and healing messages all day long?

Taking Responsibility for Your Happiness

Can you ever be happy again after you've been diagnosed with an incurable, progressive illness like MS? I'd like to think you can. For me, the answer was accepting that I deserved to be happy and understanding that it was up to *ME* to make it happen.

A parenting story I had written filled five pages in the National Multiple Sclerosis Society magazine, *Inside MS* (now *Momentum*). Our family picture graced the cover! I was thrilled! But my family's reaction was less than enthusiastic.

My husband, Dave, remarked, "You said our picture might be on the cover. You didn't say we'd be the cover!" Our 16-year-old daughter was "totally embarrassed" and our 14-year-old son glanced at the picture and asked, "Are my soccer shorts still in the dryer?"

After 3 days, the magazine was still in the same place on the table. No one had read the story, making me feel great disappointment and frustration with them.

I wondered how my family could give such little attention to what was, in my eyes, a gargantuan accomplishment. I had given up so much since MS entered my life. What were the chances of someone with my level of disability and no professional writing experience having a cover story in a national magazine? For some reason, though, my family did not seem to recognize what a great moment this was for me.

With each passing day, my depression grew. One afternoon, after crying until my eyes nearly puffed shut, it hit me! I was not going to let this disappointment pull me down any longer. I was going to take responsibility for my own happiness.

I called a local florist and ordered a basket of flowers to be delivered to my home. When the clerk asked whether I wanted to enclose a card, I said yes and dictated the following: "Congratulations! You're terrific! I'm proud of you. Love, Shelley."

Yes, that afternoon, my family and I learned an important lesson about happiness. You have to be good to yourself and celebrate your accomplishments, big and small.

I work hard to bring joy, happiness, peace, and enjoyment into my life (and sometimes this is very difficult). For example, at times, I just have to take a break from watching or listening to the news. So often the news is filled with pain and suffering that it only reinforces my feelings of helplessness and hopelessness.

Something I learned years ago from a therapist was "whatever has brought enjoyment to you in the past, try to connect with it again." I know that when I'm writing about my family, childhood memories, and experiences living with MS, I get lost in what I'm writing. It's like a vacation from my reality. I can also "disappear" when I'm on the Internet making photo books for the family or trying to learn Spanish.

Building a Support System

When people told me that I should attend support group meetings, I REFUSED to go. In fact, I didn't attend my first support group meeting until I had had MS for 10 years. Even though I was in a wheelchair, I did not identify with "those people." (Talk about denial!) No matter how old you are or what stage your MS is in, accepting your limitations, increasing disability, and an unknown future is difficult.

We can't do it alone, nor can we depend only on our family, friends, care partners, or others for all the support we need. In many cases, they are hurting as much as we are over our situation. In addition, they can't know what we're going through like others who are living with MS. Talking about how relationships with our family and friends have changed, the stress of raising kids, the inability to continue working, and the need to consider using a mobility device are only a few of the difficult issues we often need to confront.

Creating your own support system may include joining a support group, which is usually facilitated by a lay or professional leader. Meetings can include speakers; focus on a specific topic, like depression or fatigue; be social get-togethers; or a combination of all of these. Contact the MS organizations in Chapter 15 to find out whether there are support groups where you live.

Another place to find support is to contact hospitals and clinics. They often offer coping-type support groups for people with chronic illness or those who are going through life-altering changes. This kind of group will not be MS specific, but it will provide important coping strategies for living with chronic illnesses like MS.

If attending a support group is not your style or you're afraid to see others with more advanced cases, you may want to start your own small "support group" through your faith community or meet for lunch or coffee with a few selected people who are "kindred spirits" and are dealing with similar issues. Or consider connecting with people who are taking a drug you're taking (or considering taking). Patient educators, drug company representatives, and patient ambassadors can answer questions and provide important information and support.

If the everyday reminders of the difficulties you're having are too much for you, talk to your doctor. Talk therapy and medications can help with sadness, depression, and getting through difficult times. Taking an antidepressant and talking with a counselor or therapist has helped my husband and me deal with all the changes we've faced over the years. Sharing our struggles with a mental health professional improved our communication and taught us how to express our feelings in caring and loving ways. And even after living with MS for nearly 40 years, we still need a "tune up" every now and then—that is, a medication review and consultation with a therapist. Sometimes I see the therapist on my own when I "just need to talk."

Setting up a support system is up to you. In the same way, your care partner has to set up a system that works for him or her. Without proper support, living with MS is difficult at best. Take charge and create a system that works for you.

Journaling

Ever since my diagnosis in 1979, I have used a journal to record my thoughts, fears, feelings, and frustrations. I don't write every day, but I write about everything and anything—from problems I'm struggling with to interactions with doctors, from ideas for remodeling the kitchen to how I would manage when I could no longer walk or use the bathroom independently.

Writing in my journal gives me a safe place to vent, laugh, cry, worry, and share what is in my heart. After each writing session, I feel the calmness that you feel after a "good cry."

What I didn't realize when I started writing my stories and feelings was it was a way to leave a piece of myself behind. I knew that my illness was not a terminal disease. However, as you know, losing abilities can make you feel as if you are dying.

I wasn't sure how long I would live. Would I see my children go to high school? Enter college? Get married? What words of praise, encouragement, and congratulations would be missing from their lives because I was not there to utter them? What profound questions like "how will I know I'm in love?" would go unanswered? And the biggest question of all, what, if anything, would they know or remember about me?

I still write in a "journal," but now it's on the computer. And, to be honest, I've never gone back and read those first 25 years worth of entries. I know it would be too painful and sad to read how I felt back then. I know what's in them and I don't ever want to go back there. The notebooks are evidence of where I've been, how I've been tested, and how I processed my MS diagnosis. Just being there, in the file cabinet, gives me the courage to look forward because I now realize that I'm a whole lot stronger than I thought I was.

Consider writing "your story" and see what you learn about yourself.

Laughing Again

"Laughter is like changing a baby's diaper. It doesn't permanently solve any problems, but it makes things more acceptable for a while." I don't know who said that, but to me those words are a perfect analogy for life with an MS.

It is hard to laugh when you're grieving your losses, worried about the future, and frustrated by your lack of control. But I believe it is **absolutely essential** that we laugh because it makes the journey easier.

Even when I'm in the pits of my depression, I try to find some humor in the situation. One time I told Dave, "Well, when my eyes are swollen and puffy from crying, at least my wrinkles disappear!" I borrow DVDs and watch videos from the library or from friends and have found that *I Love Lucy* reruns and funny movies (*Animal House* and *Weekend at Bernie's* are my favorites) give me belly laughs.

Funny situations and circumstances are all around us. Here are a few of my favorites:

- I was explaining to my son's friend that I used to be right handed but now I'm left handed because of MS. Excitedly he said, "I know; that means, you're amphibious!"
- Then there was the time that my girlfriend, her 11-year-old daughter, and I went to the mall. My friend pulled my lift-equipped van into a handicapped-parking stall, which prompted her daughter to say, "Mom, we can't park here." From my wheelchair in the back of the van I said, "Nancy, it's OK. It's for me." We all had a good laugh and I learned that people, especially

children, don't necessarily see your limitations, even when they're obvious.

- When our son, Andrew, was in 5th grade, his art class assignment was to make a sign. Always full of "surprises," he asked the art teacher how to spell the word *cripple*. The teacher was a little reluctant and asked Andrew why he wanted to know. He replied, "I'm making a bumper sticker for my mom's Amigo" (my three-wheeled battery-operated scooter). I can only imagine the teacher's reaction, perhaps concerned that the word might hurt my feelings. Andrew reassured her, "It will make her laugh!"
- The day he brought the "bumper sticker" home he couldn't contain his excitement. Yanking it out of his backpack, he held up the 24" cardboard sign. In big bubble letters it read, "KISS THE CRIPPLE." I laughed so hard I cried; my reaction didn't disappoint Andrew. For months, we kept the sign on the front of the refrigerator and the laughter it sparked was priceless!

Self-deprecating humor or laughing at oneself is another way of finding a way of bringing laughter into your life. When I speak to audiences about strategies for living with a chronic illness, I share my personal story and add that "a strange thing happened when I lost the use of my legs and dominant right arm and hand; my mouth got bigger."

One last thought: It's impossible to cry with a smile on your face!

Getting Out

I was a master at making excuses for not going out—it's too hot, too cold, too far away, too much walking, too noisy, and so on. My favorite was "no one will miss me." It was just easier to stay home. People don't realize what an effort it takes for someone with a chronic illness to go out.

When I gave up driving, the kids were still in elementary school. Dave was wonderful and provided many rides. But by now, he was doing "my jobs" as well as his own and I hated asking him to take time off work or add one more thing to his to-do list.

I found that finding rides to school and school activities was easy. Other parents were taking their kids and kindly agreed to take mine, too. I always shared in the cost by contributing money for gas. By doing so I didn't feel as guilty asking for a ride or being part of a carpool, and people appreciated my monetary "thank you."

I don't remember exactly when I started giving myself permission to call and ask people to drive me places. But what a difference that decision has made!

Yes! It gets old having to find a driver every time I have a doctor's appointment, need a haircut, or to go to physical therapy. Many times I'll have to make five or six calls before I find someone who is free to drive me.

If I wanted to attend a meeting, event, or get-together, I didn't wait for friends to call and ask me whether I needed a ride. I called them. First, I asked people who I knew were already going whether they would be willing to drive me in my ramp-equipped van. Recently, I joined a women's group so I called the president and asked whether she knew someone coming to the meeting from my neighborhood who might be willing to drive me. She did.

My "drivers" know that if they aren't available, they have to be honest and tell me. No guilt, no embarrassment, no judgment! Many folks who aren't available will often suggest others who might be able to drive me and/or they'll say "please call me again any time."

Thankfully, people are still willing to drive my ramp-equipped van to where I need to go. However, I'm careful not to ask the same people over and over again so I don't "wear out my welcome."

After all these years, I still don't like calling and asking for rides, but I refuse to give up my life because I can't drive. There are lots of good people out there to get you where you need to go. I know, because over the years, I've gotten hundreds and hundreds of rides, met lots of interesting people, and along the way, made some new friends.

For vehicle adaptations and modification to make it easier to drive, see Chapter 13.

Helping to Find a Cure

On days when I'm feeling low or guilty for all of the things I can't/ don't do, I try to connect with a cause greater than my own, like raising funds to support MS research. Many people don't know what MS is and they've never known anyone who has it. So, whenever I have an appropriate opportunity, I tell people that I have multiple sclerosis. I'm open to their questions and am grateful for their interest.

People tend to donate more to causes when they know someone who is affected by the illness. So, when people ask you how they can help, tell them to make a donation to one of the MS organizations listed in Chapter 15 because they all fund research and provide programs and services to people with MS.

CHAPTER 3

Taking Charge—Mentally and Physically

When I was diagnosed with MS, I didn't know what the disease was although I remember being relieved that there was a name to go with my strange, difficult-to-describe symptoms. After the initial shock of being diagnosed with a serious chronic illness wore off, the reality of it began to take hold. I needed to find a way to take charge of my life and not let this disease defeat me or make me feel like less of a person.

One of the most important things that I learned was to take care of myself. This has been an evolutionary process that has taken many years and continues to this day. I believe that one day, in the not-too-distant future, there will be a cure for MS; so every day I work hard to keep mentally and physically active because I want to be in the best shape possible when that cure comes. New research, advanced technology, and discoveries have helped us better understand the mind–body connection and its importance to our total health. I encourage you to consider the tips below and develop your own strategies for taking care of yourself mentally and physically.

Memory and Concentration

When I was first diagnosed with MS, cognitive problems were thought to affect only a small number of people. Today, however, it is thought that between half to three quarters of the people who have MS have some cognitive problems, that is, difficulty with memory (acquiring and retaining), retrieving new information, concentrating and paying attention, processing information, planning, prioritizing, and word-finding.

Even though my cognitive issues are not severe—just annoying and frustrating—I still use many of these techniques and strategies to reduce my stress and maintain better control over my life.

1. If you think any of the cognitive issues mentioned earlier affect you, help is available. Discuss your concerns with your doctor, and ask to see a psychologist, neuropsychologist, or speech and language therapist, who will be able to help identify what cognitive deficits you have and how to compensate for or overcome them.

2. Write reminder notes and put them where you will be sure to see them. For example, put a sticky note on the door leading to the garage to remind you to stop at the post office for stamps or on your bathroom mirror to remind you to call a friend to wish her happy birthday.

3. Buy a small spiral notebook and a small pen or pencil that you can stick in the spiral binding and keep the notebook in your purse for when you want to write something down to remember later. You might wear a gardener's apron in the house; its generous front pockets are the perfect place to keep your notebook and pencil. Put small items in the extra pockets to keep your hands free while moving through the house or to hold those items (reading glasses, portable phones, cellphones, etc.) that you want to keep handy throughout the day.

4. Use your cellphone's address book, calendar, and notepad applications to keep your address and appointment books, notes, and to-do lists all in one place. Synchronize your phone with your computer files, so that you don't have to duplicate entries.

5. Use a timer or alarm clock that you have to physically turn off (as opposed to one that rings only once) as a reminder to turn the oven on to start dinner.

6. Have your computer "beep" to remind you to take a break and put your feet up. Program your cellphone with reminders, such

as when to take your medications, move the sprinkler in the yard, or perform certain job-related tasks, like attending a staff meeting. Or you might wear a watch with an alarm feature.

7. For tasks that have no definite ending time, put an old bracelet around your wrist when you begin the task to remind you that it needs to be finished. For example, put the bracelet on when you begin watering the yard or simmering soup in a stockpot; if you lose track of time, the bracelet will remind you to return to the task. When you're finished, take the bracelet off and put it around the outdoor water faucet or in a drawer next to the stove, so that it's ready to use the next time.

8. If it's an inopportune or inconvenient time to write yourself a note, like in a darkened movie theater or out walking the dog, take off a ring and put it on a different finger, put your watch on the "wrong" wrist, or double knot your shoelaces. That way, you'll be reminded of the task and can make a note of it later.

9. If you're "musical," create a little melody to help you remember a telephone number or sequence of steps.

10. No paper or note-taking device handy to write down things you need to remember? Try creating a word from the first letter of each item on your list. For example, C-R-O-W might mean: Call for airline tickets, Return library books, Order birthday cake, Water plants.

11. If you have trouble remembering whether you have done a task, remind yourself out loud as you do it. For example, as you leave the house and lock the door, say out loud, "I'm locking the door," and see whether that helps your memory.

12. Think over the route for the stops on your errand list before you leave home; write down the stops in the most efficient order. Consider: Is this a good time of day to be going to the library or post office? Will the drive-up windows at the bank be open? Will there be lines? Arrange the sequence of stops to make them most convenient for you.

13. Use a saddle-flap bag as a "note board." Using plain self-adhesive mailing labels, write notes on them, and stick them on the inside of the fold-over flap of the purse. Once a task or errand has been completed, peel off the label and toss it out.

14. When you are out and want to remember to do something when you return home, call yourself and leave a message in your voice mail or on your answering machine. Or call and leave a message on your cellphone.

15. If remembering and writing down numbers quickly presents a problem, keep a calculator near the phone and use it to "write down" a number.

16. To improve your ability to add and subtract numbers in your checkbook, say the numbers out loud as you work.

17. Manage your checkbook electronically.

Being accurate with numbers is a real problem for me so I use a money-management computer software program because it does all the math for you. (However, I must check the numbers I input to make sure I don't make a mistake.) The program allows me to monitor my budget, do electronic banking, and generates the information and reports I need at tax time.

Quiet Restful Activities

Fatigue is a typical problem for people with MS. I know it is for me. So finding quiet, yet mentally stimulating, activities to keep me engaged is important for my mental and emotional well-being.

Reading

18. Break in new books so they are easier to manage.

I have someone "break the spine" of a new book by opening it up and flattening the pages in several places. Books that have been well worn work better for me. I borrow them from the library or from friends, or purchase them at the used-book store.

19. Libraries offer a wide array of materials (print, large-print, Braille, audio books and e-books, magazines/periodicals, DVDs/Blu-ray, electronic games, and CDs) for patrons to borrow.

20. Most public libraries have their entire collection online and you can reserve materials from your home via the Internet. You'll receive an e-mail informing you when the books are in and ready for pickup or available to download to your tablet, smartphone, or Kindle. You can also reserve books or materials by calling your library and asking the librarian to hold them until you are able to pick them up. In some communities, they have volunteers who will drop off and pick up library materials at no charge for people with special needs. If this service would be helpful to you, ask whether it's available where you live.

21. Book stores and online booksellers like Barnes & Noble and Amazon offer a wide range of new and used library-type materials in a variety of formats for purchase.

22. With e-books and e-readers you can adjust the font size, brightness, layout, and screen orientation to make reading easier.

23. If you have a documented physical or visual disability, you may qualify for the Talking Book Program of the National Library Service for the Blind and Physically Handicapped. Some books that require a special tape player (loaned to you free of charge) are sent and returned by mail postage free. Others are available through another free library service, Braille and Audio Reading Download (BARD), which provides recorded and Braille books and magazines for residents of the United States and American citizens abroad who are unable to read or use standard printed materials because of visual or physical disabilities. Find information at www.loc.gov/nls

24. Public radio stations often have a program during which they read a chapter each day from a current novel. Check your local listings.

25. Make reading while lying in bed easier with prism glasses. You wear them just like a regular pair of glasses (they may even be worn over your existing glasses). Mirrors allow you to see a book or television screen even when you are lying flat on your back. Numerous styles are available online or where eyeglasses are sold.

26. To turn pages in a book, use the eraser on a pencil or a rubber fingertip like those used by secretaries and bookkeepers.

27. To separate pages that are stuck together, simply blow on the corner of the pages and they will magically separate.

Watching Television

28. If you juggle several remote controls for the TV, cable box, tuner, DVR/Blu-ray player, and so on, replace them with a single "universal" remote. By programming the "universal" remote you can integrate the controls into one device. Look for universal remotes, even large-button styles, online or where TVs and electronic devices are sold. There are many styles and options to choose from.

29. If you have a digital recorder, record any programs you want to see so they're available to watch at a time that's convenient for you. Locate and select programs you want to watch from the newspaper, TV guide, or Internet.

30. Keep remote controls, TV program guides, reading glasses, pens, and paper within easy reach wherever you sit by using an adjustable bed table. Or make or purchase a saddlebag-style holder with pockets to drape over the arm of your chair to hold these items.

Playing Games

31. Jumbo playing cards are available at many pharmacies or discount department stores and are easier to use than regular cards.

32. A "crooked" deck might give you a better grip as you shuffle, stack, and deal. The outward-pointing upper corner of each card makes it easier to select a single card from your hand. If you cannot find these specialty cards locally, search online.

33. To make it easier to hold cards, take an old shoebox and put the bottom of the box inside the cover. The space between the cover and the side of the shoebox holds the cards nicely.

34. Purchase a commercially available card holder. There are several types to choose from at home health stores or online. One type looks like an Oreo cookie and cards fit snuggly in between the two cookies. The cards fan out and provide a clear view of the cards in your hand. Another type is a wood platform with slots cut into the wood to hold the cards.

35. An automatic card shuffler makes it easy to shuffle up to two decks at a time.

36. Your library, senior center, or community center offer opportunities to socialize by playing cards and other games that may interest you.

37. Many popular games, such as solitaire, cribbage, bridge, Scrabble, and so on, are available online. Though you can play against others, no partner is necessary; you can play against yourself or the computer.

38. If you prefer to play any of these games with a friend, family member, or someone looking for a partner, visit your phone or computer app store to find the right game app for you.

39. A revolving game board compensates for limited reach in such games as Parcheesi, Scrabble, or jigsaw puzzles. Purchase a turntable base or use a kitchen lazy Susan for turning the game board.

40. Some games are available in deluxe versions that use all the senses to aid play. For example: The Scrabble Deluxe Edition has ridges that hold the tiles in place and a board that rotates to face the person playing the new word. Tactile overlays may be added to the tiles and board to further aid play, especially for those with visual impairments. Search online for other "adaptive (or adapted) games."

41. If you have trouble handling game pieces, substitute larger items like Lego blocks, empty plastic pill bottles, or small plastic finger puppets. To adapt game pieces like those that come with games such as Candy Land®, glue a piece of cardboard on the bottom to make the base slightly larger.

When I could no longer manage moving playing pieces, the kids or my "playmates" moved them for me.

42. Exercise your brain with crossword puzzles, Sudoku, word finds, and so on. If using the paper version in a book is too difficult, search out electronic versions you can play on your cellphone, computer, or tablet.

43. Online games, free or for a nominal charge, are available for download on your computer, tablet, or smartphone. These games can improve concentration, eye–hand coordination, problem-solving abilities, and more. Try a free version of the game to see whether you enjoy it before you purchase an ad-free version. These apps are easy to install and uninstall.

44. Memory-training games, designed by neurologists, offer a fun way to exercise your brain in many ways. AARP.org offers a selection of free games, including mah-jongg, card, arcade, strategy, word, and brain games.

Staying Active

When I was diagnosed, people with MS were advised to avoid physical exercise so as not to become overheated. With time, research has found that as with everyone else, physical activity actually reduces fatigue and provides increased strength, fitness, and a sense of well-being.

45. Before starting any exercise routine, be sure to check with your doctor and therapists for recommendations.

46. Folks with MS may want to improve their safety by participating in a "falls prevention" program offered by hospitals, clinics, senior centers, and state and local agencies. Programs are interactive and participatory. Search online for a program near you. Also consider downloading a home fall-safety checklist to help you reduce your risk of falling.

47. If you want to be more active and don't know where to start, check out the website www.ActiveMSers.org. Written for and contributed to by people with MS, the site shares expert advice on MS exercises, unbiased reviews of products, and helpful tips to be active and stay fit despite MS.

48. Yoga and Pilates are good ways to stretch, tone, and strengthen your body without a lot of impact. Look for free- or low-cost classes at a gym or local senior or community center. Your MS clinic or one of the national MS organizations may be able to help you find an appropriate group where you live.

49. Riding a bike is a low-impact activity that some with MS enjoy. If riding a bike is a form of exercise you'd like to pursue, consult your physiatrist (rehabilitation doctor) about your interest. Even if you can't ride a regular bicycle, there are seated recumbent bicycles, standing bicycles you power with a side-to-side hand/body movement, hand/arm-powered bikes, electric bikes, and three-wheeled adult tricycles to make riding easier. Search "adaptive bicycles" online. A physical therapist will be able to advise you about which bike and features would be best for you.

50. Swim at a local pool to improve your strength and mobility.

Swimming has been a great way for me to exercise. The cool water doesn't deplete my strength and the buoyancy helps support my body. I joined a university-sponsored class where kinesiology students help me into and out of the pool and with specific exercises designed to improve my strength and flexibility. It's working. I am stronger and more independent than I was before I started.

51. If you enjoyed water sports, such as kayaking or canoeing, before your diagnosis, you may continue to do so with MS. Contact your local paddle-sport store about ways to adjust your technique or retrofit your craft.

52. If you decide to join a health club, find one that has accessible facilities (handicapped changing rooms, shower seats, chair lift for the pools, etc.), convenient hours of operation, classes adapted for people with limitations, and knowledgeable trainers to help you make the most of your time at the gym.

53. Consider carrying your exercise clothes, towels, and street clothes in a (travel) carry-on bag with a retractable handle, so you can wheel them to and fro.

54. Take earplugs to cut down on the music/noise in pool or workout areas.

55. For those of you who are able to exercise more robustly, there are organizations across the United States that provide programs and opportunities to challenge you and keep you moving. By searching the Internet for wheelchair sports, you may find activities you never dreamed possible, such as therapeutic horseback riding, adaptive skiing, rope courses, skydiving, fishing, hunting, white water rafting, wilderness adventures, and more.

56. Watch the Paralympic Games or search the Internet for "disabled," "adaptive," or "para sports" to open your awareness to what feats are possible for people with disabling conditions like MS. Perhaps they'll inspire you!

Whatever activities and strategies you use to keep your mind and body active and engaged is up to you. The important message is to do things you enjoy and to stay involved.

CHAPTER 4

Medical Issues

When I was diagnosed with multiple sclerosis in my 30s, I was not prepared for the new direction my life was going to take. I think few of us are. I kept thinking this "illness stuff" would go away, or that I'd take a pill or two and be fine in a few days. However, that was not the case.

At first, I just wanted the doctors to "take care of me" and make me better. I thought they knew better than I did. How naive I was! It didn't take long for me to realize that that's not the way things worked.

I learned how important it was (and still is) for me to become a partner in my medical care. We are responsible for our own health care and it's in our own best interest to speak up, get involved, and be heard. Learning to stick up for myself and being my own advocate has given me back some of the power and control that MS has taken away.

In this chapter, you'll find tips and strategies that, I hope, will give you the strength and encouragement you need to ask questions, ferret out information, make informed decisions, and take charge of your medical care.

Where to Start

1. Learn as much as you can about MS; its types, treatments, medications, and current research. My friends and family members also did research and collected information. We shared information and learned together. It gave us something positive to do.

2. No matter what doctor or health care specialist you see, be completely honest.

If I'm not forthcoming, my medical team will not have all the information they need to treat me properly. I try to focus on all the symptoms I'm having, no matter how minor or silly they might seem. Some completely unrelated concerns were my first symptoms of MS—I couldn't run as fast as I used to and the fingers on my dominant right hand felt "slowed/stiff" when I fingerspelled to my deaf students.

3. Choose doctors who you can relate to.

I have learned that a health care provider's bedside manner is extremely important. If a particular doctor doesn't treat me with respect, listen to me, or see me as a whole person—a wife, mother, daughter, writer—I find someone who will.

4. It is important that you choose one doctor to be your primary care physician—someone with whom you feel comfortable voicing your concerns and fears, whose office is convenient for you, and whose staff is attentive to your needs. If you are able, try to find a doctor who has experience in treating people with MS. You and your doctor will be partners in your medical journey so you want someone you can relate to.

5. If you are on Medicare or Medicaid, make sure to ask any new doctors whether they accept assignments; if you don't ask you may be surprised with a big bill.

Record Keeping

6. All public and private health care providers are required to provide electronic medical records (EMR), a computerized medical records system designed to share records between providers and the patient. Your personal medical file helps you keep track of your current prescription medications, as well as over-the-counter drugs and vitamin, mineral, and herbal supplements; past illnesses; surgical procedures; and family history. Via the Internet, you can review previous medical test results and procedures, make medical appointments, and communicate with your doctors. To learn more about obtaining and maintaining your medical records, contact your health care provider.

7. At times it may be helpful to keep a notebook, log, or diary and to document changes in your condition, new symptoms, and questions you have for your health care team.

8. Keep a current list of all medications (dosage, strength, how often you take them), including over-the-counter medications and supplements you are taking, in your wallet or cell phone for instant access anytime you need that information.

Doctor Appointments

9. When scheduling a doctor's appointment, ask how much time you will spend with the doctor. Depending on the reason for the visit, you may be scheduled for as little as 5 minutes or as much as an hour. If you have a lot to talk to the doctor about, schedule a "consultation" appointment so the doctor will have enough time and be unhurried.

10. When making an appointment or scheduling a test, tell the scheduler whether you will require any special help—for example, assistance undressing or getting onto the examining table.

11. If you are using paratransit (transportation for people who cannot access the public transit system because of their disability), to and from your appointment, explain that you have a scheduled ride with paratransit and that after your appointment you must be at the door waiting at a predetermined time or your ride will leave without you. Ask whether there is a better time of day to see the doctor so that he or she will be on time. Once you arrive at your appointment, remind the receptionist about your scheduled pickup time.

12. If your energy level is highest in the morning, try to get the doctor's first appointment of the day. If you schedule your appointment first thing in the morning or immediately after lunch, you will be

less likely to have to wait to be seen. Early-evening appointments may afford a more leisurely office visit.

13. If you are anxious to see the doctor soon and there are no open appointments, ask to be put on the "wait list" and to be notified if someone cancels. Don't be afraid to call the clinic every few days to ask about any cancellations.

14. Before leaving home for your appointment, call your doctor's office and ask whether the doctor is running on schedule. The receptionist may suggest you come in a little later instead of spending so much time in the waiting room. Regardless of the wait time quoted over the phone, it's always wise to bring a book or reading material with you.

15. Consider bringing a friend or family member with you to appointments. Between the two of you, you will remember more of what the doctor has to say about your condition and treatment options. You might use your smartphone or a digital recorder to record your visit so that you can review your doctor's explanations and answers to your questions after you get home. At the very least, you, or the person who accompanies you, should take notes of what your doctor says.

16. If you don't understand completely what the medical professionals are saying, ask for clarification. Don't hesitate to state, "I'm not sure I understood that. Would you explain it again?" Or, "Do you have written materials for me to take home and read over?"

17. When you meet with the doctor, clearly and briefly describe your concerns without embarrassment. Be specific. Share important events in your personal, professional, and social life. Difficult times and stressful events may affect your health and how you take care of yourself.

18. If you have questions or concerns about something and are not sure it warrants a doctor's appointment, contact the doctor's office and leave your questions for the nurse, nurse practitioner, or physician's assistant. When someone calls you back, share your concerns. These support professionals will speak with the doctor and relay your questions and either they or the doctor will get back to you.

19. Follow your doctor's advice. If you have trouble following your treatment, talk to your doctor. Don't quit. Finding the right treatment program often involves trial and error. Be patient.

20. Stick to proven remedies recommended by your doctor. Avoid "miracle" treatments hyped in the media or through direct marketing.

21. If your doctor orders a test, ask when the results are expected. If you don't hear from the doctor in a timely way, call and ask about the results. If you feel you need a second or third opinion about a medical condition and/or care, follow your instincts. Second opinions are now standard practice and your doctor(s) should understand your desire to get all the information you need to make informed decisions.

Prescription Medications

22. When medication is prescribed, ask your doctor about the best time to take the medication, possible side effects, and what you should do if problems arise.

23. Be sure to ask your doctor whether generic drugs, which are less expensive than brand-name drugs, may be used to fill your prescription.

24. Ask your doctors whether they have any samples or can prescribe a 1-week sample dose so you can try the medication to see whether it works, or there are any allergies or unpleasant side effects before you purchase a month's supply.

25. Make sure the drug prescribed is on your insurance company's formulary and find out what your copay will be. If it's an expensive drug, see whether there is a lower cost alternative or a payment plan.

26. Ask whether it is possible to safely prescribe a higher dose and cut the pills in half.

27. Ask your clinic staff or pharmacist to see whether you qualify for any prescription-assistance programs.

28. Make sure you and your family know how any prescribed medications work, what the side effects are, and which side effects to call the doctor about. Do not take any other medications, including nonprescription products, without checking with your health care team.

29. If you select one pharmacy to fill your prescriptions, you will have a complete record of your prescriptions in one place. The pharmacist will be able to check that a new prescription does not adversely interact with a medication you are already taking. If you travel, consider using a pharmacy with a national network of stores so you can get refills while you are away.

30. Develop a working relationship with your pharmacist; pharmacists work with medications every day and are often the most knowledgeable about how drugs might affect your body and can inform you about any possible side effects, contraindications, or undesirable interactions that could occur among new prescribed drugs, over-the-counter medications, and even certain foods like grapefruit juice, coffee, milk, or alcohol.

Taking Medication

31. Start a new medication as early in the day as possible. If you have an adverse reaction, it will be easier to reach the doctor.

32. To remember to take a medication first thing in the morning, put the pill bottle in your slipper. Before you can put your slippers on, you must remove the pill bottle.

33. If you have trouble removing childproof tops from your medication bottles, ask your pharmacist to replace them with regular covers. However, if you have children in the house, you will need to be especially careful to store your medications safely out of reach.

34. If you still have trouble opening prescription bottles or you find the print too small to read, ask for your prescriptions to be put in large-size, easy-to-open containers with large-print labels.

35. If you have trouble reading the prescription medication materials the pharmacy provides with your prescription, ask the pharmacist to include a large-print copy. You may also use a magnifying glass to help you read the small print.

36. Once you get home with a new medication, note on the label what the drug is for to remind you to use it only for the prescribed condition.

37. A Talking Rx pill bottle, designed for those with low vision, allows you, your pharmacist, or a family member to easily record a spoken message with instructions on how to take the medication. To hear the dosage instructions, you simply press a button on the cap. You will find these devices online.

38. Be sure to find out what you can do to make taking your medicine easier. Is it all right to crush or break your pills—or even dissolve them in water? Is a more palatable option available, such as a liquid or granules? It is risky simply to break open a capsule or crush a tablet. Many are sustained-release formulations, which are designed so that the medicine seeps into your bloodstream over many hours. To release the entire dose all at once could increase your risk of side effects or even be toxic.

39. Never use household tableware to administer medication, especially for children, for whom exact dosage is important. Always use an oral dropper, cylindrical dosing spoon, syringe, or plastic medicine cup, all available from your pharmacy, and be exact in your measurements.

40. If you use a medicine dropper to give liquid medications by mouth, release the liquid slowly into the cheek. Be careful not to point the dropper into the throat, which might force the medication down the windpipe.

41. If you have difficulty swallowing a pill or tablet, ask whether you can place it in a teaspoon of pudding, applesauce, or mashed banana to make it easier to swallow. If you still have trouble, ask your doctor about an alternative, such as taking several smaller pills rather than one large one.

42. Chew a small piece of bread until you are about ready to swallow it. Then put the pill in the mass of bread in your mouth. Once you close your mouth, drink some water, and swallow the food with the pill inside.

43. Fill a plastic bottle with water. Put the pill on your tongue and close your lips snugly around the opening of the water bottle. Put your head back and take a drink of the water using a sucking motion to swallow the water and pill.

44. Place the pill in a spoon with honey or a dollop of peanut butter. Drink some water before and after you take the "spoonful of medicine" to lubricate the throat.

45. If the act of physically picking up a pill is difficult, lick your finger and tap the pill. It will stick long enough to put the pill in your mouth.

46. Ask your pharmacist the best way to store medications—a high-humidity bathroom cabinet usually is the worst place to put it.

47. To make keeping track of your medications easier, use a seven-compartment molded-plastic pill dispenser that has individual snap-lock compartments with a hinged lid and a letter for each day of the week on top. Some models come with multiple compartments for morning, noon, and night. Weekly pill dispensers are readily available at pharmacies or online.

48. If you are taking multiple medications, create a dosage schedule that you carry with you and check off each dose as you take it.

49. Use an alarmed-reminder pill organizer. Fill the organizer, then set up to four alarms per day to remind you when to take your medication. You can also use a digital watch with an alarm feature or program the alarm on your cell phone.

50. Save time and energy by ordering prescription refills several days in advance and have the pharmacy mail them to you.

51. If your medications are delivered by a courier service and you need extra time to get to the door when the delivery is made, notify the company sending you the medication when you place your order. Some companies will accommodate your request by having the delivery person wait until you answer. To have medications delivered when you aren't home, you may need to sign a release form to allow the delivery person to leave the package in a designated place.

52. When getting a prescription refilled, ask the pharmacist to put the expiration date on the front information panel for each prescription. Prescriptions are packaged from large bottles that contain great quantities and often are marked with an expiration date that is not transferred to monthly prescription refills.

53. Mark on a calendar the days when medication should be increased or decreased.

54. Drink water when taking medications.

When I took a medication that required that I drink a large quantity of water each day, I put an empty gallon container next to the sink and every time I drank a glass of water, I poured an equal amount into the gallon container. When the container was full, I knew I had drunk the prescribed amount of water.

55. Many medications, as well as head and neck radiation, can cause dry mouth. Saliva is important to maintain healthy teeth and gums and aids in swallowing, digestion, and the ability to speak normally.

56. Chewing gum (preferably sugarless) will stimulate saliva production; there are also over-the-counter dry-mouth products available. If the condition persists, consult both your doctor and dentist.

57. Dispose of medications properly. Most communities have a drop-off site for unused or expired prescriptions. Do not flush them down the toilet; they may end up negatively affecting wildlife or drinking water.

The Hospital

58. Take along all the things you need from home to be comfortable, like a favorite pillow, a reacher, amplified telephone receiver, favorite music, and so forth. Make sure to take along the phone numbers and addresses you may need, including family and friends, as well as your next-door neighbors', landlord/property manager, employer, medical supply company, and so on.

59. Be sure that everyone who treats you washes or sanitizes his or her hands.

60. Hospitals routinely scan your wristband before administering any treatment or medication. However, mistakes do happen so speak up if you think something is not as it should be. Learn to recognize the medicines you are supposed to receive.

61. Before undergoing tests and procedures, ask about the purpose, risks, and possible discomfort. If possible, talk with other people, perhaps members of your support group who have undergone similar tests, treatments, and procedures so that you can have an idea what to expect.

62. Be clear about your needs.

When I have the preprocedure/preoperative interview, I explain that I have difficult-to-find veins so I always need an especially skilled person to put in the IV. Otherwise, getting the IV started could cause serious delays in their schedule. I also mention that I'm unable to walk, transfer, or change positions without assistance. I want the staff to be prepared and have the equipment and manpower they need to help me.

63. Hospitals are busy places and it's difficult to get needed rest. If you do not want to be disturbed, turn off your phone and put a "Resting, Please Do Not Disturb" sign on your door. Then, if hospital personnel enter your room to pick something up or drop something off, at least they will do so quietly.

64. If the location of the room or your roommate prevents you from getting your necessary rest, you have the right to request a transfer to another room.

65. If you're not up to having visitors, be honest and tell your friends and family when they call.

When I've been hospitalized, I had the nurse post a note on the wall above my bed that read: "Please limit visits to 20 minutes."

66. Find out what time the nurses' shifts change, so that you can ask for anything you need at least an hour before, when they aren't busy writing up reports and performing other change-of-shift duties.

67. In an emergency, if no one comes when you press your call button, use the phone and call the nurses' station directly. (Get this number from the staff or from contact information cards usually given to immediate family.)

68. Hospitals have patient advocates—hospital employees whose job is to make sure your concerns are not overlooked. Use this resource if you are concerned that you are not receiving adequate care.

69. If you are hospitalized, it is best to designate one person in the family to be the one in contact with your doctor. That way, one person is asking the questions on behalf of the family, which avoids duplication of effort by both your family members and your physician.

70. Sometimes family and friends can help with nonmedical procedures such as feeding, repositioning, transferring, walking, and assisted coughing. Ask your nursing staff what is possible.

71. Before an emergency or scheduled hospitalization arises, be sure to have an Advanced Medical Directive and Durable Power of Attorney for Health Care in place. These documents will allow your family or designated health care agent to make important medical decisions should you be unable to do so.

72. Before you are discharged, your hospital social worker or discharge planner will want to know about your home situation and can inform you about community services and resources you may not be aware of that may help make the transition to home easier. You will need to discuss how much care you need and who is best qualified to help you. Will someone check up on you at home on a regular basis? Will you need home health care services? If you will need medical equipment for short-term or long-term use, the discharge planner can help you make these arrangements as well.

Managing Your Home Health Care

73. If you have just been released from the hospital, take the phone number of the nursing station from the floor where your room was located. Once you're home, if you have questions in the middle of the night, you will have someone to call who can allay your fears or tell you to come in for emergency treatment.

74. If you want to keep friends and relatives apprised of your progress, but don't want to be disturbed, let your voicemail or answering machine provide the information. Each day record a new message updating the medical report or send an update by e-mail or group text message.

75. As you recover from an exacerbation, your child may be "recovering," too. It's frightening for a child when Mom or Dad is sick. Watch for signs of stress and provide a little extra TLC to reassure your child that you are OK and that you are working to get better.

76. Post important medical information on the refrigerator, like a list of medicines you have to take and at what time or foods and liquids you should not have. Friends, family, and helpers will find the information helpful.

77. Keep a list of important telephone numbers near each telephone, such as those for police and fire departments, electric and gas companies, poison control center, family doctor, dentist, and neighbors. Include your home address and phone number on the list in case a neighbor or health care provider needs to tell emergency personnel.

78. Keep your cell phone with you at all times. In emergencies or national disasters, your cell phone may not work if cell phone towers can't handle the load or there is a massive power outage. Even if some cell phone towers have generators, their power may be time-limited. Landline phones generally work during power outages because they do not require electricity to function. A landline phone may be especially important for folks who often require access to emergency services.

79. If you need emergency medical assistance, make sure someone can inform the rescue workers of your condition and your special physical needs.

See Chapter 9 for more Home Safety Tips.

Authorizations, Denials, and Appeals

80. When dealing with your clinic, HMO, a hospital, or insurance company, ALWAYS keep notes of who you spoke with (have them spell their first and last name), when you spoke with them (date and time), and what was said. This way if there are questions later, you will have a record of your discussion to both remind you of the details and back you up in case of a discrepancy.

81. If your clinic, HMO, or insurance company denies treatment or won't authorize services that you feel you need, there is a grievance process. Do not accept a denial when you know the treatment will help you. Take charge! Get your doctor's support in writing and appeal the original decision as many times as necessary to get what you need.

Additional Medical Resources

82. The National Library of Medicine is the world's largest medical library and offers information about diseases, conditions, treatments, and wellness. Learn about your prescription drugs and over-the-counter medicines, including side effects, dosage, special precautions, and more. All the information is presented in easy-to-understand layman's terms (www.MedlinePlus.gov).

83. The Medicine Program's Patient Assistance Program is a free service to help you apply and qualify for the appropriate Patient Assistance Program(s). A patient advocate works with you and your doctor, and the prescription drug manufacturers help you obtain your medication free or almost free-of-charge (www.themedicineprogram .com).

It's easy to get overwhelmed with all the information and decisions you have to handle when you have an MS diagnosis. I hope that the suggestions and ideas provided here offer you the support and encouragement you need as you become an active participant in your health care.

CHAPTER 5

Family and Friends

Having friends has always been important to me, but never more so since learning that I had MS. Frankly, I don't know how I would have survived without my friends. But friendships can get "complicated" when you have a chronic illness.

In the months following my diagnosis, I noticed a change in some of my friends; they stopped calling me and inviting me to participate in their get-togethers. They just "drifted away." I think some were impatient with the extra time it took me/us to do things. Some didn't want to be bothered by my special needs. Or perhaps I was a subtle reminder to them that bad things can happen to good people. It was a sad and painful time for me.

Looking back, I can say that the friends who "walked out" made room in my life for new people to walk in. My new friends are people who love and accept me, limitations and all.

I've also come to understand that friends often pop in and out of our lives over many decades. To me it wasn't/isn't so much about my MS, it's more about the stage of our lives, that is, work friends, playgroup moms, exercise buddies, book club members, and so on.

It's also true that people have different interests and talents and I've learned to capitalize on that. Some enjoy cooking so we get together and cook cauldrons of chili, soup, and stew, which we divide up for our freezers. Some like doing errands and going out to lunch. Some make me laugh even when I don't feel like it. One person has volunteered weekly for nearly 20 years. She fixes my lunch and stays to water plants, open mail, send out birthday cards, wrap presents, and help me in the bathroom and into bed. No one could ask for more special friends.

I now understand and accept that everyone has his or her own way of doing things. When my friends help me in the kitchen making lunch, for example, some clean as they go. Some wait until after we've eaten to clean up. Some wipe off the stove and countertops without thinking. Others need to be reminded. Rather than being critical or complaining, I remind myself that it's the friendships that are more important to me than a spotless kitchen.

Making New Friends

It was difficult to make new friends in the beginning. Because I had cut back on everything just to get through the day, I didn't have the energy it takes to establish new friendships. But over the years I discovered some techniques that have helped bring new people into my life.

1. Focus on what you enjoy, like reading, swimming, gardening, playing cards, woodworking, and so on. Then, consider finding a book group, craft, bridge, or swim club, and so on. Spending time with people who enjoy the same things you do provides an opportunity to establish new friendships.

2. Take a class. If making a weekly commitment is too much, join a group that meets once a month. Can't take a class that lasts for months or has homework? Take a 2-hour (cooking, writing, art, etc.) class. Not only will you get out of the house, but you'll meet like-minded people and potential new friends.

3. Invite people over to your house. Whether it's a regularly sched-uled activity to play cards, watch a video/sporting event/favor-ite program or an occasional neighborhood get-together, host the gathering at your home. Then you won't have to be concerned about bad weather, transportation problems, or difficult-to-get-to locations.

4. Ask your friends to come over and bring a friend, especially if that friend has an interest or talent that you'd like to develop. Learn how to use a computer, send e-mails, make greeting cards, do desktop publishing, and so on. Most people enjoy showing others their hob-bies and helping them get started. (Think how good you would feel, if you were asked to teach someone about something you enjoy.)

5. Can't clean the house for guests? Straighten up the meeting room and the bathroom and close all the other doors. Remember, you're trying to establish new relationships, not prove you're a super housekeeper.

Use the Internet to Make New Friends and Keep the Old

6. Facebook, MS support groups, chat rooms, and blogs are just a few of the ways you can connect with others who have MS. Don't just focus on MS groups. Explore familiar topics, things you want to learn more about, or just surf around until something catches your interest. Then connect with some of those folks.

7. Reconnect with old friends, especially those you enjoyed at another time in your life. The Internet can help you locate childhood friends, college roommates, a special teacher, or former neighbor.

Keeping Friendships Strong

I remember calling a relative to tell her about my MS diagnosis. Her response was to tell me that I must have a deep psychological need to be sick and that if I went into therapy and dealt with the underlying issues that were "making me sick," I'd be healthy again. Can you imagine? I was shocked and hurt by the insinuation that my medical problems were "all in my head."

That was many years ago and during the intervening years I have learned that I'm not the only one who has experienced the hurtful and insensitive words of others. My guess is that you have, too. The question is, "Do we let the negative words, actions, or feelings of other people eat away at us? Or do we let them go and move on?"

Here are a few of my thoughts for keeping friendships strong:

8. Look at what might be behind the person's words or actions. Were they said or done in jest? In the heat of an argument? Or did the person make an offhand comment? Sometimes people don't think

before they speak or act and have no idea how what they have said or done has caused such a hurtful reaction.

9. Evaluate how well you know and how much you care about the person. If the person is someone you have known forever and have a history with, share your feelings and tell the person how the words or actions affected you. Starting with an "I" statement, like "I felt . . .," "I thought . . .," "I needed . . .," will open up a conversation. Starting with a "you" statement, like "You always . . .," "You said . . .," "You think . . .," will either shut down the dialog or take your interaction in an argumentative direction.

10. Limit the amount of time you spend with negative or toxic people. Don't feel guilty when you make excuses for (not) getting together, cut telephone calls short, or screen your calls.

In the early years of my diagnosis, my friends wanted to protect me from "bad news." They thought I had enough to deal with and stopped telling me about their health issues, a difficult child, an impending divorce, and problems with aging parents. I understood their concern and told them that, good or bad, I wanted and needed to be kept in the loop. I still wanted to be a caring and committed friend.

It isn't always easy being my friend. There are still times when I pull back and isolate myself, especially when I'm going through a difficult time or transition. I always try to be upfront and honest with the people in my life and thankfully folks have come to understand when I "need some space." I was grateful that my friends respected my needs and didn't take my "pulling back" personally. They know that I will reach out and re-engage when I'm ready.

11. Let people help you.

When people say, "Let me know how I can help." I do. My friends have picked up things for me at the grocery store, taken books back to the library, picked up prescriptions from the pharmacy, and more.

12. Try to keep in touch with friends and relatives who have moved away or live out of town.

I began sending a "winter letter." I started the tradition the year I was diagnosed with MS. I wanted to tell people the news and share how we were managing. Over the years, the letter has taken on a life of its own and people have come to expect my yearly update. I'm still writing the letters but now I use the computer and send the letter out via e-mail.

Healthy relationships are a vital to overall health and well-being, especially when you have MS. It's imperative that we feel loved, respected, supported, and encouraged by the people in our lives.

CHAPTER 6

Marriage

On August 27, 1979, our lives changed forever; it was the day I was diagnosed with multiple sclerosis. Our lives had been so perfect. Dave and I had been happily married for 10 years. We had two beautiful preschoolers, great jobs, and a home in the suburbs. Life couldn't have been better.

When I was diagnosed with MS, I remember how Dave and I held each other, fighting back the tears of pain and anguish. I remember the questions we were too scared to ask. And I remember how the dreams we had for the future disappeared right before our eyes. We had no way of knowing the challenges that would lie ahead. Our marriage and commitment to each other would be tested time and again. Would we be among the 50% of the marriages that ended in divorce when a spouse becomes chronically ill or disabled?

Today, it's hard to believe that our marriage has survived nearly 50 years and prospered despite the challenges we faced. How did we beat the odds? Why has our marriage survived and thrived?

I'm not sure I know. But it made me start thinking. I decided to ask Dave why he thought we'd made it and he said, you tell me first. So here's my response.

Shelley's Story

When I was first diagnosed, we knew very little about the illness and neither of us knew anyone who had it. We had to learn together. Our love and respect for each other and our open and honest communication made all the difference.

During those early years, I tried to handle everything as though nothing had changed. I just cut back a little and stopped going to evening activities. I wanted to save my energy for Dave and the kids. I tried to rest while Dave was at work so that I'd be up physically and emotionally when Dave got home. He didn't like coming home to find me in bed.

It seemed that every day I lost a little something and it made it especially hard on our marriage. My fingers were weaker, my legs were stiff and "heavy," and oh, that awful fatigue! I was so frustrated and scared: What would I lose next? Like most men, Dave wanted to fix it. But he couldn't fix this so he was frustrated, too.

Many times our feelings and emotions of anger were over-whelming and we'd yell at each other to vent our frustrations. On more than one occasion Jamie begged us to stop fighting. She was scared that we were going to get a divorce. And Dave, no matter how angry he was, always came to my aid when I needed his help.

Over the years my physical condition continued to deteriorate. I tried hard to keep a positive attitude and remain optimistic. But by the end of each day, I'd be in tears. Tears of frustration and disappointment were just too strong to squelch. And then I'd feel guilty for dumping on Dave. He was sad, too. Sometimes he held me when I cried. Sometimes he gave me the space I needed and let me cry alone.

It couldn't have been easy for Dave to watch me being subjected to all sorts of medical procedures and treatments: plasmapheresis, chemotherapy, megadoses of prednisone, ACTH, hyperbaric oxygen, and intravenous methylprednisolone, just to name a few. (None of the currently available treatments and therapies had been discovered back then.)

The side effects and mood swings were often worse than the MS. The hospital stays that kept me away from home were hard on Dave and the kids. Thankfully, our family and friends helped Dave shoulder the responsibilities.

Whenever I felt I was losing the emotional battle, I'd see a psychologist. Dave was always supportive and probably relieved that I could vent my frustrations on someone else. Since I started taking antidepressants more than 30 years ago, the mood swings have leveled out. Around the same time, Dave was diagnosed with clinical depression and started taking antidepressants, too. Taking advantage of advances in medicine helped us both cope better.

Another way we coped was to simplify our lives. I pulled back from all but essential activities and commitments. I'd do the more sedentary child-rearing activities like reading, playing board games, and supervising the kids dress, clean up the toys, do school work. Dave did the more active things like giving the baths, playing soccer and baseball, and teaching the kids how to ride bikes, ice skate, roller skate, and so on.

The kids were wonderful blessings, but they sure did present challenges! Dave and I took our parenting responsibilities very seriously. Suffice it to say, sometimes the kids brought us closer together and other times they caused great conflict.

Dave and I felt it was important to take time out from our parenting duties and spend time together. We'd always had an active social life and he wanted that to continue. He didn't like it when I used my MS as an excuse to stay home and he worked to accommodate my needs. (For example: I ALWAYS needed a 2-hour nap midday.)

I knew it was hard on Dave that my MS was such a disruptive force in our marriage. I tried to make accommodations and find creative ways to say thank you for his love and support. For an anniversary one year, I "kidnapped" Dave and took him on a mystery overnight trip. For 3 days prior, one of my friends drove me to Dave's office so I could drop off a little gift (a rose, chocolates, and champagne with two glasses) and each gift included a love note. I arranged for my mom to babysit the kids, cleared Dave's work calendar and made the reservations at an out-of-town hotel. I gassed up the car and had money for the getaway. I didn't tell Dave the destination, but gave him directions. All he had to do was drive the car. We had a great 24 hours to ourselves. He loved it and so did I!

And then, as a way of expressing my appreciation for "waiting on me" for the 3 months I was in bed healing a stage 1 bedsore, I made him a HUGE promise.

I hereby promise that for the rest of our lives, I will not complain, roll my eyes, or otherwise say one disparaging word about you watching any kind of sporting event involving a ball, including the Major League Baseball Network and all its programs; hundreds of games on Major League Extra Innings; replays of games you recorded after seeing them live;

classic games—baseball, football, or basketball; Sports Center; Plays of the Day ... (I was too nauseous to name more.)

I will not make any comments regarding your channel surfing or restrict your ability to watch any of the preceding programs in the bedroom, where you can recline comfortably on your electric bed. No matter how many innings, overtime periods, or instant replays there are; my lips are sealed!

I honor my promise to this day.

Normally, things went pretty well. But there were the inevitable emergencies that Dave had to handle with minimal help from me, like the time the dishwasher overflowed and the kitchen floor was flooded with suds. Dave had to clean up the mess while I sat on a chair and watched. Or the time the freezer door was left ajar and Dave had to do marathon cooking to salvage the food. My contribution was to sit at the kitchen table and look for simple recipes we could use to cook the defrosted foods. Or the time a water pipe burst in the basement and Dave had to do all the cleanup himself.

Even though Dave's been blessed with almost limitless energy, I tried to take things "off his plate" whenever I could, like sending his shirts to the cleaners, so he didn't have to stand at the dryer waiting to pull the shirts out. I planned meals and made out grocery lists so we had well-balanced meals and Dave only had to shop once a week. I arranged carpools so Dave didn't always have to drive me or the kids. I shopped by phone to locate items we needed and Dave just had to pick them up. (Remember, this was before the Internet and shopping online.) I know these were such little things in comparison to all that he was doing, but it was the best I could muster, and he appreciated it.

I also tried to give Dave permission to have a life of his own. I didn't want him to stop playing softball, tennis, or riding his bike. I wanted him to be able to go to work without worrying about me and the kids. I turned to relatives, friends, and neighbors, and arranged for daily helpers so he knew the kids and I had the help we needed. He didn't always like me asking other people for help. I think he thought it made him look weak or less than capable. Sometimes we'd argue about it. But I'm convinced that our marriage couldn't have survived without my reaching out and asking others for help. No one can do it all!

I've also worked very hard to make a life of my own, separate from Dave and the kids. I wanted to remain interesting and have experiences that I could talk about. I was tired of talking about how I felt, what the doctor said, or how long I napped. I wanted more! I keep as busy as my energy and stamina will allow.

For nearly 30 years, there wasn't much I could do for myself physically. I had only minimal use of my left hand. I wasn't able to use the bathroom by myself and I needed help getting into and out of bed. Every night, I disturbed Dave's sleep, waking him to help turn me over. And then, in the past few years, for some unknown reason, my MS has stabilized and I've gained back some physical abilities. (Could it be from exercise, physical therapy, counseling, mindfulness, prayers, or miracles? Maybe it was a little of everything. I don't know.)

Thankfully, Dave makes me feel as though he needs me as much as I need him. In fact, sometimes I think he doesn't even realize that I'm disabled. I've come to realize that the little things I do really do make a difference. They keep us communicating and connected. When I listen, support, love, respect, understand, appreciate, and care, I'm telling this wonderful man how special he is to me. And maybe that's why our marriage has lasted.

David's Story

I remember Shelley coming to my office that August afternoon and how upset she was. I was concerned, but didn't really know what that diagnosis of MS meant, so I suppose you could say I minimized the situation. After we both talked to the doctor, we still didn't have a clear picture of what the future would bring, and I didn't want to worry unnecessarily.

In the very beginning, I think the hardest thing for me to handle was that she was tired all the time. We always had to schedule a rest time for her no matter how active or sedentary our plans were. If she overdid it, which happened frequently, she'd be in tears. Nothing but a long nap helped. I hated it when we had to cancel activities and disappoint the kids, and I didn't like leaving her home to rest and taking the kids to the park, parades, shopping, and so on, without her. I know she didn't like it either but she rarely complained.

I guess I could never totally understand what she was going through. Even though she would tell me that she felt herself getting a little weaker every day, I couldn't see it. It took a few months for the weaknesses she described to show up in a way that I could see, like not being able to braid Jamie's hair or not being able to run after Andrew.

I wasn't prepared for the unrelenting pace with which she was getting worse. As she slowed down and cut back on the physical aspects of our family life, I started doing more and more. At times I was angry because I felt that once I took over doing the laundry, for example, she abdicated responsibility and let me take on that chore as if it was now my job. Sometimes I felt she didn't even care if these household chores got done. Yet at times it seemed she had the energy and stamina to do the things she wanted to do.

I've always had much more energy than Shelley did and over the years I've learned to accept that Shelley needs a nap or downtime every day. And, to her credit, she listened to me and now makes an effort to become more involved in our day-to-day life and household activities.

The first few years I think we managed to function pretty normally. But, 5 or 6 years after her diagnosis, when she could no longer drive the car or walk from one end of the house to the other, I really began to worry about the future, and the stress took its toll. I developed stomach problems and lost 20 pounds. After lots of tests, the final diagnosis was clinical depression. (I certainly got a taste of what it was like for her dealing with doctors, medical procedures, and the vast unknown.) It was not fun!

Even from the early years of our marriage, we've had a loosely formed "division of labor." I like doing the finances and investments, which I did before Shelley got MS. When the kids were in school and need helped with school projects that involved/difficult assignments, I was usually the one to handle those tasks. Shelley was and is the emotional "caretaker," and the one who the kids, now adults, still rely on. We always make big decisions together and I appreciate her attention to detail when we buy appliances, vehicles, furniture, and so on. She's practical and wants to be sure she can use, operate, or manage any product we purchase.

Growing up, both of our families were social and enjoyed entertaining so we have always tried to follow that same family tradition. We have a wide variety of friends and Shelley always handles our social calendar and entertainments. When we have parties and holiday gatherings she creates and organizes the menu, asking friends to bring a dish to pass, creates a shopping list for me, helps me in the kitchen, and sets the schedule so everything is ready to serve at the same time. I don't mind doing most of the physical work as long as Shelley is there guiding me.

A major highlight in our lives was a surprise party that she planned for my 39th birthday. More than 100 family members and friends came from all over the country to celebrate. Shelley, with help from family and friends, pulled it off and I was totally and completely surprised!

It's been so long since she was in the hospital that I can hardly remember it. Yet, I don't think I'll ever forget when she was hospitalized in Milwaukee for extended periods. It wasn't easy for me to juggle everything in Madison, 90 miles away. Thank goodness my parents came and helped me with the kids, who were only 10 and 8. It wasn't easy for her to handle these treatments, but she always went in with great hope and optimism. When these treatments didn't stop the progression of the MS, she was really down. It hurt to see her so terribly disappointed.

I don't know whether I would have been able to handle all the medical aspects of having a chronic illness as well as she did—all the medications that changed her appearance, made her nauseated, caused mood swings, sapped her energy, and gave her headaches. And then all the spinal taps, myelograms, intravenous (IV) injections, and so on. It was pretty bad. At times I felt frustrated and irritated having to deal with the medical stuff. Thank goodness we had good insurance, or I would have felt completely overwhelmed.

Some other ways I found to deal with the tension of having a spouse with MS was to do some physical exercise. I walk, ride my bike, do yoga, and play tennis. I make time to do things I enjoy, like watching or attending sporting events, managing my fantasy baseball team, staying a part of my monthly poker group, and remaining active in my leadership role at our temple.

It was hard living without hope. I understood why, after trying everything mainstream medicine had to offer, she looked to nontraditional treatments for help. The trip to Germany and the every-other-day IV injections I gave her, the costly acupuncture treatments with vile-smelling teas, and the bee stings I gave her 3 days a week that caused huge welts are the things that stick out in my mind. It was crazy! I guess I wanted to believe, like she did, that SOMETHING had to stop the disease from progressing.

I wouldn't be telling the truth if I didn't admit that I got angry and felt resentful because I had to do everything, especially when there were so many things going on at work and at home. I still get irritated when her requests for help interrupt what I'm doing, like working in the yard, exercising, or watching a ball game. These days, I'm really annoyed when she wants my help doing things that I don't think are a high priority, like when we had a Fourth of July party and she wanted floral arrangements on all the tables. I didn't want to be bothered.

I didn't mind when she asked people to help her with lunch, take her to an appointment, or help her write notes to friends and relatives (before computers and e-mail). I didn't like it when she asked for help for things I felt I should be doing, like driving carpool, doing grocery shopping, and making meals.

However, the things that sometimes "get to me" (e.g., when Shelley would go to great lengths to stay independent) also are her strong points and, in some ironic way, are loveable, admirable qualities. For example, it has always amazed me that Shelley is able to boldly ask friends, neighbors, acquaintances, even people she doesn't know for help when I'm not around. When she needs help getting lifted into the passenger seat of our full-sized van and her driver is not able to help her, she's gotten help from the chef at a restaurant where she was eating lunch, the Bobcat guy landscaping the next-door neighbor's yard, and the young man collecting carts in the parking lot of a big-box store, to name a few.

Yes, I wish we could be more spontaneous and could just pick up and go. It gets old planning and making special arrangements to accommodate her needs. Yet, Shelley is always looking for the positives that we have in our lives. Undaunted by challenges and situations, Shelley is always positive and says, "We'll figure it out."

Instead of the active lifestyle we had before MS, we spend time with family and friends "hanging out," playing games, going to plays, concerts, classes, movies, sporting events, and more. And, I appreciate that whenever I want to spend time with my buddies playing tennis, going sailing, attending a sporting event, and so on, Shelley encourages me to go and finds a friend to get together with while I'm gone.

One of the things we both enjoy is a good laugh. We are funny and tease each other regularly and I love that she appreciates my dark humor. As just one example: I used to tease Shelley's friends who came to drive her to appointments/events that if they kept her for more than 2 hours, they shouldn't be surprised if her bags were sitting on the driveway and the ramp was gone.

I do worry about the future. At some point, I'm not going to be able to help her physically like I do now. Our retirement years are going to be very different than that of our friends. But we have traveled a tough journey together, and I have great faith that we will find our way through this stage of our lives together, too.

So why did I stay? I don't know. I never thought our life together was that bad. I feel lucky to have her as my life partner. She's the mother of my children and I couldn't imagine my life without her. We are there for each other no matter what. We enjoy being "empty nesters," and to this day, we love when the kids and grandkids come for a visit, but we love it when they go home and it's just the two of us again.

In spite of the serious disability she lives with each day, anyone who is with her for a short time forgets about her disability and sees the wonderful, warm, and caring person she is. I love her very much for all that she does despite her severe limitations. I respect her for her accomplishments (author of seven books and hundreds of articles and columns) helping others coping with chronic disabling conditions like MS. And most of all, I love and respect her for not giving up because if what happened to her had happened to me, I would have given up long ago.

CHAPTER 7

Sexual Compatibility and Intimacy

In this book, I've been very open and honest about living my life with the complications and frustrations that multiple sclerosis creates. Several areas that remain to be approached are the following: (a) How should a person with MS deal with a dating relationship? When and how do you share that you have MS? and (b) sexual compatibility and intimacy. How do you deal with the physical and emotional challenges chronic illness presents?

First, the issue of dating. It is important to remember that Dave and I had been married for 10 years when I was diagnosed with MS. Frankly, if I had been diagnosed with MS while I had been dating or in a relationship, I don't know how I would have handled disclosing my MS. I'd probably ask my medical professionals or folks from national MS organizations for advice and support. Once I had gathered information and ideas and processed what I learned, I'd trust myself to handle the situation in a way that was right for me. If the person I was seeing had a problem with my news, I'd rather know sooner than later that there were "red flags" that could affect a long-term relationship.

Now, let's talk about sexual intimacy and compatibility when an individual has MS. I know it's a very important topic that even "normal" couples deal with. I believe that all couples deal with sexual compatibility issues from time to time. Whether it's because of an illness, age-related changes, or the stresses of life, it's normal as our relationships change and evolve. Although Dave and I feel comfortable sharing some broad advice, we agree that our own experiences with these topics are a little too personal to share.

With that being said, I can offer the insights and understandings we have gained over nearly 50 years of marriage. Perhaps the most important point is that you must be able to communicate with each other. Honesty on the part of both people is imperative. Waiting until anger and frustration come to a boiling point is never good. In addition, both people have to listen to and acknowledge what the other person is saying. It's not easy!!! I know from personal experience that having a positive, loving relationship with your partner takes hard work from both of you. If your relationship is troubled and filled with conflict, having a chronic illness like MS will put additional stress on your marriage and will impact your intimate relationship.

In terms of sexual intimacy and compatibility, Dave and I have experienced many of the issues that couples dealing with MS confront. For us, some of the topics that we've had to deal with from time to time were and are (my) fatigue, the effects of medication on my body, stresses in our lives, clinical depression and anxiety, and the never-ending frustration of living with the issues that I've written about in this book.

Dave and I had to learn to be honest with our medical professionals, often bringing up the subject of intimacy to our doctors. I found it interesting that they never asked us about our sex life or whether we had any concerns that needed to be addressed. If you have any concerns, talk to your primary care physician, neurologist, or someone from your health care team with whom you feel comfortable sharing your concerns. Ask them to explain how your MS can have an impact on intimacy and sexual compatibility. In addition, ask about the effects medications and therapies can have on your desire and libido, as well as your self-esteem and body image. There are dozens of resources you can refer to for more information on all the topics related to intimacy and MS. Here are a few:

- www.NationalMSSociety.org
  - *Website search topics*: "Living well with MS," "family and relationships," "intimacy"

- ○ *Publication*: *Intimacy and Sexuality in MS* by Rosalind C. Kalb (2012)
- ○ *Online learning class*: Intimacy: Enriching your relationship
- Multiple Sclerosis Society of America (www.MyMSAA.org) Search topics: "Intimacy," "love," "sex," and "relationships"
- Divorce Busting (DivorceBusting.com): Offers help for sexually troubled marriages
- The Marriage & Family Health Center (www.passionatemarriage .com): Offers sexuality education and therapy programs
- American Association of Sex Educators, Counselors, and Therapists (AASECT; www.aasect.org): Offers information and referrals for certified sex therapists
- Sex and MS (www.WebMD.org): Offers suggestions for maintaining intimacy with MS
- Everyday Health online (www.EverdayHealth.com) search topics: "Intimacy," "sexual intercourse," "low libido," and more
- www.Sharecare.com search topics: "Feelings and relationships," "relationship challenges," "sex and relationships," "good in bed"
- The Sinclair Intimacy Institute (www.sinclairinstitute.com): A catalog of adult sex education videos
- A Woman's Touch—Sexuality Resource Center (www.sexuality resources.com)

MS presents challenges in every facet of our lives and some challenges are more difficult than others. Please don't be embarrassed or afraid to confront any difficulties you may have. Intimacy is an important part of being a human being. I hope the resources and suggestions I've made will help you find answers and the help you may need.

CHAPTER 8

Being a Parent

Being a parent has been the biggest challenge in my life while living with multiple sclerosis. In this chapter, I share dozens of real, personal stories and examples from over 4 decades as a parent—most of those years with MS. I believe my experiences provide valuable insights into what it's like for parents with MS. Looking back, I feel that this information would have provided an invaluable guide for me and made my job as a parent easier and less stressful. I hope you find the strategies, how-to tips, and techniques helpful as you make your own parenting decisions and create your own parenting style.

My husband, Dave, and I found our first HUGE issue was what do we tell the children about my illness? When I was diagnosed, our children—daughter Jamie and son Andrew (5 and 3 at the time)—were so young. However, even though they were so little, they "knew" that something bad had happened—Mom cried a lot, and Dad, Grandma, and Grandpa talked in hushed tones. Outgoing little Jamie didn't want me to leave her sight, and happy-go-lucky Andrew began sucking his thumb, something he had stopped doing months before.

One night Dave and I gathered our courage and told the kids that Mommy had an illness that the doctors didn't know much about and there was no medicine to make Mommy better. Jamie's first question was, "Mommy, are you going to die?" (At just 5, she could ask such piercing, perceptive questions.) That night I cried myself to sleep thinking that MS had robbed my children of the carefree childhood they deserved. And I vowed to try to keep our world as normal as possible.

Although I am not an expert in child-rearing techniques or child development, I'd like to think that I've learned a few things. Today, our son and daughter have turned out to be loving, caring, responsible adults with spouses and children of their own. Being their mother was worth every sleepless night and gray hair they gave me. I am very grateful that I now have validation that my MS didn't ruin their lives. If anything, perhaps it made them stronger, more compassionate, and more capable than many adults with less dramatic and less stressful upbringings.

One reason our family has survived my MS is that we are open and honest with each other. Questions get answered no matter how difficult or embarrassing. My husband, Dave, and I won't pretend that nothing's wrong. When there's a problem, we talk about it and search for answers together; sometimes we involve the children in our discussions. We believe that we must work together if our family is to survive. It wasn't anyone's fault that I got sick; it merely meant that we needed to be there for each other a little more often.

So, how did I manage parenting all those years? How did I cope? What do I know now that I wish I'd known then? Read on to find out.

Parenting 101—General Concepts and Strategies

1. Kids are born with personalities. Some are quiet and laid back from the moment they're born. Others are busy, busy, busy, all day and night. Children assert themselves at a very early age and it's our job as parents to adjust.

2. All children go through normal, developmental stages—temper tantrums, being afraid of thunderstorms, nightmares, and so on. If the behavior lasted longer than 6 to 8 weeks or got *significantly* worse, I consulted the pediatrician, teacher, other mothers, or community resources to learn whether my child's behavior was within normal limits.

3. Children often regress before they make a leap in development. Little ones may want to be carried everywhere just before they start walking. Kids may become homebodies before they start wanting to sleep at a friend's house.

4. At our house, every day between 4 p.m. and 5 p.m. was the "arsenic hour." Why? Because children are tired, cranky, and irritable and so are the parents. A healthy snack helps everyone!

5. Children want some control in their lives, so pick your battles carefully. What difference does it make if your 3-year-old wants to wear ridiculous outfits to preschool? Who cares if your middle schooler sprays her hair pink, or your teenager wants to wear sandals with his Prom tuxedo? (Take a picture. One day, you'll all get a big laugh.)

6. Give the kids lots of opportunities to learn how the "real world" operates and how their actions/inactions have consequences. What happens if you don't put your dirty clothes in the laundry basket, fail to hand in classroom assignments, forget to return library books, forget school permission slips, or to put gas in the car? Enduring these experiences today is the cheapest price they will pay to learn valuable lessons; as kids get older, the price goes up. After all, the price a 10-year-old pays for not locking up his bike and having it stolen is not as high as the price he might pay for not locking the car at night and having it vandalized or stolen.

7. When you have two or more children there always seems to be someone who demands extra time and attention.

8. Consider "incentives" (i.e., bribery). For example: If you want kids to pick up their rooms, have them do it before they go out to play or use technology. Don't expect their rooms to be spotless; however, do expect some semblance of order. When you're not up to an argument and can't stand looking at the mess, close the bedroom door.

9. One of the phrases that I used throughout the parenting years was "feel free to . . ." "Feel free to go out and play, as soon as your room is picked up." "Feel free to watch TV after you've finished your homework." Or "feel free to use the car after you've cut the grass." This technique works with kids of all ages, but it's especially effective with teenagers.

10. Kids learn valuable lessons through trial and error. Fight the temptation to jump in and take over, even if you can buckle their shoes, make the salad, or straighten the bedroom faster and more efficiently. In addition, when you make comments like, "You're not doing that right." "What's taking you so long?" "I better help you," you're undermining your kids' self-confidence and self-esteem. Just stand back, be patient, provide verbal guidance and encouragement.

11. Kids also learn valuable lessons from their mistakes (especially if you can avoid saying "I told you so").

When Andrew was 11, he had to sell raffle tickets to help defray the cost of playing Little League. He collected nearly $75 and left it lying around his room. (I bit my tongue and didn't say a word.) It's still unclear how it happened, but $25 disappeared. When it came time to turn in the money, Andrew had to use his birthday money to replace the missing $25. Needless to say, it was a very painful lesson. Two months later, when the school sponsored a pizza sale to purchase new playground equipment, I was tempted to step in and take over, but I didn't. I wanted him to know that everyone makes mistakes and what's important is that making mistakes is how people learn and grow. He must have learned his lesson because he's never had another problem handling money.

Communication

12. When parents don't share information, children conjure up all kinds of fears—some of them are worse than the reality—and, we end up "teaching" them to keep secrets and withhold information from people who love and support us.

13. Giving voice to and sharing that you're sad, angry, or frustrated is OK. When you're upset about something, tell the kids why. "I'm angry with myself for being sick." "I'm sad because I just ordered my first wheelchair." "I'm frustrated because I can't braid your hair anymore." Acknowledge their fears and give them permission to be angry and frustrated with MS and its presence in your family.

14. When we're positive and upbeat, our homes are more relaxed. I learned that when I cried and "lost it," the kids would clam up; they didn't want to upset me further. When we needed help

coping with the stress that MS was creating in our lives, we sought out help through the family doctor, an MS clinic/organization, the school, or our faith community.

15. Listen to your kids; sometimes they say things that we need to hear.

Jamie was 12 when she told me: "Stop yelling at me! You're not mad at me. You're mad at the MS. Go take a nap and you'll feel better when you wake up." She was right. I wasn't angry with her. I was frustrated, weary, and exhausted from trying to keep up, do what I used to do, and follow through with plans that I had made. Oh, how I wanted to be "normal" again!

16. It's difficult having MS and when things pile up and get over-whelming, I go to my room and cry until the only thing I can do is to fall into a deep exhausted sleep. When I wake up, I feel calm and peaceful, ready to regroup and face the world.

17. Sometimes the kids (inadvertently) get the wrong idea and think that they caused our illness. As parents, we MUST remind our children that they are not responsible for our illness. Having MS is not anyone's fault; no one is to blame.

18. Model appropriate adult behavior. No matter how old kids are, they are always watching us and recording our behavior.

Dave and I try to avoid yelling, swearing, giving each other the silent treatment, even screaming at other drivers, and so on. We recognized early on that one day our kids might say, "You say/do that! Why can't I?"

19. As much as you love your kids, do not let them take advantage of you. We MUST show, by example, that people have a responsibility to take care of themselves!

20. When we "misspeak," I believe we should acknowledge and apologize for it.

Sometimes, with the children I had an inappropriate knee-jerk response— let's say to an accidentally spilled glass of milk. (If a friend had spilled the drink, I would not have had the same reaction.) "Kids" of all ages have accidents. A better response would have been, "Let's get the mop and get this cleaned up." Whenever I misspoke or "behaved badly," I'd apologize to the kids for "overreacting" and we'd talk about how I might handle the situation differently next time.

21. We must help kids acknowledge and understand their own anger and frustration with our illness. It's perfectly normal for them to get angry or resent the effects our illness has on them.

There were times when Jamie and Andrew hated having to come home after school to help me. I'd tell them, "I understand you'd rather go to a friend's house than come home and that I'd probably feel the same way if my mom had made me come home. Being angry with me and this illness is OK." Kids need to know that having these feelings doesn't make them a bad person. It's also important that kids know they are not responsible for me, nor do they need to be "the man or lady of the house."

22. Sometimes WE need to make changes in the way we talk and interact with our children.

Knowing that I could "only change myself" helped me a great deal as a parent. I stopped making demands, sarcastic remarks, lecturing, and asking questions like: "How many times have I told you to …?" or "Why can't you listen/understand/remember?" I thought I'd feel angry if someone talked to me like that, so I began beginning my sentences with "I"; I felt nicer, and the kids responded positively to the change.

I tried hard to be consistent, but there were plenty of times when there was "an uprising" that I was too tired or too angry to handle. At those times, I'd send the offending person(s) to his or her bedroom until I could calm down and think clearly. I certainly didn't want to impose a punishment that would be impossible to carry out or too severe for the offense.

23. When kids behave inappropriately, disobey you, lie, and so on, consider asking them what they think a fair punishment should be. Sometimes kids are tougher on themselves than you would have been. And they aren't nearly as angry with us for the punishment they receive.

24. Ask your children for their thoughts and opinions. Then listen. Don't judge. Just acknowledge and consider their ideas. Let them be an active participant in family discussions. Whenever appropriate, involve them in making decisions—everything from what we should have for dinner to where we should go on vacation. All of us need to feel valued and respected and that includes children.

25. Being an authoritarian parent is not in our kids' best interest.

The world has changed since Dave and I were children and we realized so must we. If we wanted to have a good relationship with our kids, we had to bury the belief that we held all the power. As they grew, we learned to stand in the wings and support the decisions they made. When we did that, we sent the kids a powerful message—"I know you can handle this situation. I trust you. You're a competent, capable person." It's a complex world with complex problems and we wanted them to be prepared to live in it.

26. It's not easy having a parent with a disability; so let the kids know that their help and understanding are appreciated. Give the kids compliments. Tell them how proud they make you. Say "please" and "thank you." We all like to know that our efforts are valued.

27. Kids are very sensitive about how parents talk to them in the presence of their friends.

I'm careful not to embarrass Jamie or Andrew in front of their peers. Just as I hope they won't embarrass me in front of mine. I save my editorial comments for when we're alone.

28. Treat your children with respect.

Throughout their growing up, we treated Jamie and Andrew with respect, even when they were showing their less-than-perfect sides. I tried to react like a rational adult. Sometimes I was successful, sometimes I wasn't. My motivation was the Golden Rule, which I learned as a child: "Treat people the way you would want to be treated" because one day your children will be in a position to treat you as they were treated. That's a sobering thought.

Fostering Independence

29. When the kids help you, accept the level of help they are able to provide. They may not do things to your satisfaction, but the job will be done and, as the kids get older, their skills and abilities will improve.

30. Teach children how to do things and provide lots of opportunities to practice.

31. At each age, we involved Jamie and Andrew in everyday household activities. At 3, we expected the kids to carry their dishes to the sink after a meal. When they were a little older, they helped us get ready for company. Under our guidance, they learned how to use the washer and dryer, read road maps, and organize and prioritize their school assignments. In high school, they knew how to drive downtown alone, balance their checkbooks, and manage school and part-time jobs.

Realities for Parents With MS

32. For children who have a parent with a chronic illness like MS, there are concerns and worries children their age wouldn't be expected to have.

Jamie, for example, worried that I would die. She worried about tornadoes and how I would get down to the basement if the sirens went off. She wanted to know who would take care of me when Dad couldn't lift me anymore. Would I have to live in a nursing home? Andrew asked me if I thought a girl wouldn't want to marry him because he had a mom who was disabled. Clearly, these were not issues of concern to most children.

33. It's scary for kids of all ages to have a sick parent, especially at times when there's a flare-up. I learned much later that sometimes the kids were afraid to ask questions or talk about my MS because they didn't want to upset me or make me cry. At times like these, it's important for our kids to have someone (relative, family friend, clergy, school counsellor, etc.) they can talk to if they have questions or worries they think will upset you.

34. Kids also need reassurance that "no matter what" they will be taken care of. Talking about who would be there to help them (grandparents, relatives, and close family friends) is essential to lowering their stress and worries.

35. If you are in the hospital or undergoing tests or treatments, tell your child's teachers (school psychologist/counselor) to watch for signs of stress or behavioral changes and to alert you if they have concerns.

36. Things that you think are watershed events don't always register with your child in the same way.

The first time I tried (and failed) to use my first scooter at the local zoo, I had a complete and total temper tantrum when Dave brought the scooter to the passenger-side door for me. I demanded to be taken home, NOW. I was too embarrassed and mortified that I now needed a scooter. The kids tell me they have no memory of the incident.

37. Sometimes the results of our illness cause our children pain. One time, when I came to school to vote, a classmate of Jamie's saw me walking and asked Jamie if I was drunk. When I no longer had the strength and dexterity to braid Jamie's hair, we had it cut short. The next day, at school, a friend told Jamie that her hair looked ugly and asked why in the world she got it cut. I ached for the pain my MS caused.

38. I admit it, when I was having a "bad day/episode," the TV was often a babysitter. Today, with all the technologic devices available, you have a whole new world of "babysitters" to keep the kids engaged when you can't depend on your head and heart to agree with your energy and stamina.

39. Whether it's watching a video together, playing an educational game on the iPad, using YouTube videos to learn how to do something, or researching information of special interest to one of the children, I'm spending quality time with my grandchildren. I love how we are making memories and learning new things from each other.

40. When kids have friends over to play, things can get "out of control," especially on days when we're not feeling up to par. In desperation, you may need to send everyone home. Afterward, take the opportunity to calmly talk with your child about what happened and how you might avoid the situation in the future.

41. Whenever I could, I tried to put a positive spin on my MS and disability. "Aren't we lucky to have this disabled parking permit so we can park close to the door?" "Aren't you lucky that I have my Amigo® scooter so you can sit on my lap when you're tired?" "Aren't you lucky (that I can't drive), because you have a car at your disposal when you need to get to and from work?"

House Rules

Because of my increasing disability, our family needed to create some house rules. It was the only way we could function.

42. First, there were our hard-and-fast, non-negotiable rules: No playing with matches. No running into the street, and so on.

43. Equally as important were the rules governing good moral and ethical conduct: No lying, cheating, or stealing.

44. We also had rules that kept us organized. A grocery list and pencil hung from the refrigerator door. If you finished or used the last of anything, you put it on the list.

45. Dirty clothes had to be put in your hamper if you wanted your clothes washed. Clothes left on the floor were not picked up and washed. (The kids learned to use the washer and dryer at an early age.)

46. Bedrooms were their own domains.

Yes, they had to pick up their rooms, but I couldn't waste my energy fighting with them over the meaning of "picked up." Fortunately, a favorite babysitter mentioned how messy their rooms were and because Jamie and Andrew were so embarrassed by her comment, they began doing a better job of straightening their rooms.

47. Schoolwork and chores came before recreational and social activities.

48. We also had rules governing mealtime and meal preparation. Mealtime has always been a family affair and everyone pitches in, even our guests. I teased that I was the "sidewalk-snoopervisor." We had one, non-negotiable rule: NO ONE LEAVES the kitchen until everyone leaves. It is amazing how helpful and efficient even young children can be. When they got a little older the rule was expanded. "Everyone eats meals, so everyone is involved with meal planning and preparation." Jamie, age 9, and Andrew, age 7, were proud of themselves when guests watched them cutting vegetables with a sharp knife and using the stove to make grilled-cheese sandwiches.

49. When friends were invited for dinner, they were expected to participate in the preparation and cleanup of the meal.

When Jamie attended the University of Wisconsin—Madison, her roommates would often come for dinner. One of her roommates remarked that our family was like "The Cleavers." Pretty funny, given that I was very severely disabled, unable to stand, walk, or get into or out of bed myself. Clearly, we were not that iconic "perfect family." Yet, her observation may have been related to the fact that everyone took part, no matter what needed to be done.

50. Be creative and make house rules that work for your family. Learn how other families add structure and organization to their homes.

A few years ago, a cousin told me that she and her husband were having trouble getting their three children (elementary and middle-school age) to bed at night. The parents were exhausted and did not like the nightly hassle, delaying tactics, or the early-morning nagging to get the kids out of bed. Their creative and successful solution? The parents told all three children that they could stay up as late as they wanted. However, they were responsible for getting up and ready for school the next morning without any parental involvement. Risky? Yes? But it worked for them.

Chores

51. In the early years, I encouraged the kids to be "Mommy's Little Helpers" by helping me dust, fold laundry, set the table, pick up the family room, and so forth. However, I began to realize that I was giving them the wrong message. By calling them "Mommy's Little Helpers," I made it sound as if I was the one who was responsible for doing certain tasks in the house and that they were in fact, helping "me" with "my" jobs. Instead, I started saying, "It takes everyone's help to have a nice place to live and it's important that we all pitch in to get the chores done." It was a subtle but powerful distinction.

52. Encourage children to be creative problem solvers no matter what their age.

53. When Andrew was 5 I was no longer able to collect and carry the laundry baskets from each bedroom down to the basement where the washer/dryer were. Instead of beating myself up emotionally for yet another thing that I could no longer do, I asked Andrew, who was too small to carry even one basket, whether he knew how we could make the task easier. His solution? He took a belt and used the holes/openings in the baskets to join two baskets together. Then he took another belt and used it to connect a third basket. Then he took a rope and tied it to the first basket. Once the rope was secure, he threw the rope over his shoulder and pulled the baskets behind him down the hall, through the kitchen to the stairway to the basement. Then, he stood at the top of the stairs and threw pieces of laundry down to my waiting arms. Instead of feeling sad and frustrated over needing more help, darling little Andrew made me laugh.

54. Dave and I rearranged where we kept kids' toys and games to give them more independence. Boxes, shelves, and containers were within easy reach. (No climbing necessary.) The added benefit to having a place for everything was that when the kids were done playing, they could put their toys away. They were often slow or reluctant to clean up, however, there was no TV (or bedtime story, or snack) until things were put away.

55. Under my guidance, they learned to use knives, the stove, the microwave, and blender. The fact that my hands were too weak to do most tasks meant I couldn't jump in and take over. With words of encouragement, they HAD to do the task themselves. These experiences gave them confidence to tackle more complicated kitchen and household tasks as they grew. In high school, for example, their friends were always impressed that both Jamie and Andrew knew how to plan a meal, follow a recipe, and time it so that all the dishes came out at the same time.

56. To avoid hassles and arguments, I was careful who I asked to help with which chore. Jamie, for example, was the organizer and liked to keep things tidy, whereas Andrew liked fixing things and doing more active chores.

57. I needn't have worried or felt guilty that having responsibilities and doing chores put too much pressure on the kids. They are now parents themselves and, as a grandmother, I am now enjoying watching these lessons play out in the next generation. Perhaps I was a pretty good "real mom" after all.

Discipline and Sibling Rivalry

58. Discipline and sibling rivalry are issues parents face daily.

Because I didn't want Dave to become the only parental figure, I had to find new ways to deal with conflict within the family. I couldn't get sucked into battles because it was energy depleting. I had to encourage the kids to talk it out and find solutions to their disagreements. I warned them that if I had to get involved they wouldn't like my decision.

59. All children jockey for position and all parents have experienced small children bickering and whining over whose toy is whose. Even when they were young, we all would brainstorm and come up with lots of ideas, some silly, some serious, to solve disputes. The final solution was a compilation of all our ideas and was agreeable to everyone. "Fighting" over who got the front seat in the car, which restaurant we went to, or what movie to watch, provided lots of opportunities to practice their abilities to listen and find compromise.

60. When a cookie, a piece of gum, or a candy bar needed to be divided equally, tempers often flared. One half always seemed bigger than the other. To avoid this problem, we let one child divide the item "in half" and let the other child chose which half he or she wanted.

61. As children grow, conflicts often get physical, with pushing, shoving, or just "touching."

When I didn't know who "started it," I sent each child to a neutral corner. While in the corner, they were expected to talk to each other until they could work out a solution. At first, they'd yell and scream, making ridiculous threats like, "I'm never letting you out of your corner for a hundred, billion years," or "I'm never going to play with you again." When they realized I wasn't going to help them solve their problem, they began talking to each other. When they reached a solution, each had to give the other permission to leave the corner.

62. When kids are old enough to babysit each other, conflicts can arise.

The first time the kids babysat for each other, there was bickering and tattling when we arrived home. We solved the problem by saying that they would both get paid to babysit if they were able to get along while we were gone. If one tattled on the other, no one got paid.

The Early Years—Birth to 10

Those early years taught me many valuable, lifelong, parenting lessons. Perhaps they'll help get you started on creating your own set of "survival tips."

63. Giving kids choices is an easy way to "finesse" control. "Do you want the Hot Wheels cup or the Star Wars cup?" "Are you going to wear a sweater or jacket to school today?" "Do you want to take a bath or a shower tonight?"

64. We gave the kids opportunities to make their own decisions. We let them choose which pair of shoes to purchase, the style of their haircut, and, within reason, what outfits they wore to preschool/public school.

65. We encouraged independence by letting them turn on the TV, pour the milk, and carry their plates to the sink.

Because my MS had weakened my hands and arms, I remember giving our children opportunities to put on their shoes and dress themselves even when they were young. It always took extra time and lots of patience on my part, but I was proud of them for trying and appreciated their efforts. They liked doing it themselves and, as they grew, they became more adept at the tasks.

66. Have a schedule and you will limit the drama while adding structure to your family. I don't think we could have survived without schedules. Meals, for example, were generally around 7:30 for breakfast, lunch was around noon, and dinner was between 5:30 and 6:30. There was always a small snack (fruit, string cheese, yogurt, etc.) around 4:00.

67. When the kids napped in the afternoon, I did too. To keep from being disturbed, I hung a "We're Resting" sign on the front door. (When their friends were too young to read, I used a picture of a sleeping baby on the sign and explained to their little friends what that sign meant.) Adults and children learned not to ring the bell and disturb us when the sign was present. After the kids gave up their naps, we all had a quiet time, a 45-minute rest period, after lunch during the summer and on school vacations. I got in bed to rest and the kids read or played quietly in their rooms.

68. When I needed extra downtime, I hired a neighborhood child as a "mother's helper" to come over after school to play with the kids. I was still in the house should they need me; however, I was resting or having a "quiet time."

69. Have nightly rituals to help kids wind down at the end of the day.

70. We always had snacks before bedtime. Then, once the kids were in their pajamas with brushed teeth, they could watch TV for half an hour. There was story time after that and then it was lights out. They learned that delay tactics would mean shortened or missed TV or story time.

71. We used the family room as the playroom. I could keep an eye on the kids and the "mess" they created was contained to one area.

72. To eliminate the effort of packing the kids up and taking them out, I invited another mom and child over. These moms were also my friends and knew of my health problems. We'd sit where we could see the children and visit while they played. Before they left, everyone helped clean up.

73. From the time the kids were very young, we played board games while I reclined on the couch or lay in bed. When I couldn't reach or grasp the game pieces, the kids moved the pieces for me.

74. I can't remember exactly when I made the rule that after 9 p.m., I was off "Mommy duty." If the children wanted my help with schoolwork, a class project, or any activity requiring brainpower, it had to be before then. After that, my brain was fried.

Bathing

75. When bathing young children, consider using liquid soap in a pump dispenser to keep soap from slipping from your hands.

76. If your child doesn't like to be bathed, he or she may feel more secure sharing a bath with you. Or you might sit on a lawn or shower chair inside your shower stall and hold your child on your lap.

77. Keep bath toys consolidated by putting them in a hanging mesh laundry bag after bath time is over. Hang the bag on the faucet in the bath so that the water can drain out.

78. If you feel that you might have trouble lifting a slippery or heavy child out of the bathtub, drain the water out of the tub and dry the child first. Then dress him or her in a cotton T-shirt and lift the child out of the tub.

79. Purchase terry-cloth bathrobes for your children and put them on immediately after bathing. It's an easy way to dry children off.

Changing the Sheets or the Baby

80. To make changing the bed at night easier, we always layered the sheets by alternating waterproof underpads (bed pads, sheet protectors, Chux) with contour crib sheets. Then, if there is a wet bed at 3 a.m., simply lift off the sheet and the underpad and the next sheet with underpad is dry and ready.

81. In a diaper bag, keep a clean outfit for your toddler in a resealable plastic bag. The outfit is all in one place and you can seal the soiled garments in the empty plastic bag.

Dressing

82. It's safer to dress a child on the floor rather than on top of a changing table, a bed, or on your lap.

83. It is easier to dress young children if they hold a raisin or piece of dry cereal in their hand. Closed fists make it easier to get hands through sleeves.

84. Slip a sock over your child's hands and arms before putting on a snowsuit. Leave the "mitten socks" on and you'll eliminate the gap between the mitten and the cuff of the sleeve.

85. Teach young children how to put on shirts, jackets, and sweaters without your help. Have the children lay the garments on the floor with the collar nearest their feet, all the front buttons unbuttoned, and the inside of the garment facing up toward the ceiling. Then have them bend over and put their arms into the armholes and lift the garment up and over their heads. Children will be proud of their accomplishment, and you'll be thrilled because they don't need your help.

86. Show your kids how to line up buttons with the appropriate buttonhole by dressing in front of a mirror.

87. Involve your children when you purchase their clothes. (Even an 18-month-old has strong opinions about what he or she likes to wear.)

I've learned that imposing my taste and not including the kids in clothing purchases is an area ripe for conflict. Also, as soon as they are able, insist that their selections be easy to put on and take off independently.

88. Each evening before bed, have kids select their clothing for the following day, offering choices that you can live with. "Do you want to wear the teddy bear sweatshirt or the rainbow sweater?"

89. Getting kids to try on clothes to see if they still fit was always a problem.

Here's what we did: We had a style show. (If grandparents or relatives are available, invite them for the performance.) As the kids tried on the clothes, they selected jewelry, shoes, and hats to go with each outfit. Have your camera ready!

Shoes and Socks

90. Sprinkle a little cornstarch on the bottom of your child's feet before putting on socks.

91. Putting shoes on a wiggly toddler is easier if the child is "trapped" in a high chair.

92. Children have an easier time putting on shoes that fasten with Velcro®. Help them to select shoes they can put on and take off by themselves.

93. To teach a child how to put the right shoe on the right foot, mark or tape the inside of the right shoe only.

Mealtime

94. Put a plastic mat under your child's high chair for easier cleanup.

95. Purchase plates with a high outer edge or lip or with suction bottoms. They prevent food from sliding off the plate.

96. It is easier to spread peanut butter on a slice of frozen bread than on a slice at room temperature. The frozen bread does not tear, is easier to hold on to, and defrosts so quickly that by the time your child gets to the table, it is ready to eat.

97. Buy whipped butter and cream cheese; they are easier to spread than the standard variety.

98. Let children serve themselves with the understanding that they must eat all the food they take.

99. Create a special "kid shelf" in your kitchen and stock it with healthy foods in predetermined portions. Kids enjoy the control and you'll be able to monitor the types and amount of snacks your child is eating.

100. Save energy at the grocery store by letting kids help retrieve things from the shelves. Depending on their ages, give them hints to the products you want—the box with white flowers on it, the 12-oz bottle, the spaghetti sauce with mushrooms and garlic, and so on. Grocery shopping can be a game that provides a fun learning experience.

101. Getting enough sleep was always a problem for Dave and me.

To stay in bed a little longer on weekend mornings, we helped Jamie and Andrew get their morning snack ready the night before. They poured some of their favorite cereal into a bowl with a snap top. The bowls and spoons were left on the kitchen table and a lightweight, easy-to-pour, plastic pitcher of milk was in the refrigerator on a shelf they could reach. When they got up, they could eat their breakfast and watch TV until we got up. It was a win–win for everyone.

102. Little hands will find it easier to hold onto a drinking glass if you place two tightly wound rubber bands around the glass an inch or so apart or give the child a drinking glass with a bumpy exterior.

Health and Safety

103. Give young children liquid vitamins/medication when they're sitting in a high chair. If the medications have the potential to stain, give it to them when they take a bath.

104. To look down a reluctant child's throat, use a lollipop as a tongue depressor.

105. To prevent a toddler from going outside unsupervised, fasten bells above exterior doors. When the door opens, the ringing bells will get your attention.

106. When children are old enough to answer the door, they need to remember to ask, "Who is it?" and wait for an acceptable answer before they actually open the door.

107. If you want to keep young children out of a certain room, child-proof it by putting a sock over the doorknob and winding a rubber band tightly around the base of the knob, to keep the sock from being pulled off. The door can be easily opened by adults who can squeeze the handles and turn them, but the socks just slide around the knob in a child's grasp. To make the doorknob's diameter even bigger and harder for children to turn, use padded doorknob covers.

108. If your kitchen drawers have handles (rather than knobs), an easy way to childproof them is to slide a yardstick (straight up and down) through the handles.

109. When you're out and about, especially in stores and crowded public areas, it's easier to keep track of the kids if you dress them in bright easy-to-see colors.

Activities

110. When we could arrange it, the kids were involved in indoor and outdoor sports (ice skating, gymnastics, tennis, soccer, swimming, etc.). Because I was no longer able to drive, I asked other parents if they would have room in their carpool for my child. People were amazingly kind and inclusive.

111. When traveling, teach kids how to pack their backpack and explain how they can only take what they can carry.

The Middle Years (10–14)

The middle years were a time of daily contradictions that kept me reeling. By this time, I'd had MS for 5 years and was severely disabled. I never felt well and was ALWAYS home. I often felt like I was an embarrassment to the kids.

When their friends were over, I laughed too much or I didn't laugh enough. I talked too much or I was being mean and ignoring them. Jamie thought my clothes were "old looking," but the next day she wanted to wear one of my sweaters to school. I often felt I couldn't do anything right.

My self-esteem was dwindling with the loss of my physical abilities, but it was comforting to learn that other (healthy) parents were dealing with the same pre- and early-teen mood swings I was. None of it had anything to do with MS or my disability.

112. Kids want and need more independence.

Being exposed to new friends and families in middle school gave the kids new experiences and with it came their desire (i.e., demand) for more independence. I had to find solutions that worked for us. For example: When severe fatigue meant I didn't have the stamina to go to the mall, I gave 11-year-old Jamie the credit card to go shopping with her friends. She brought her selections home "on approval." Once home, she'd put on a fashion show and we'd decide together which items to keep and which ones went back.

113. Teaching kids responsibility.

Dave and I encouraged the kids to take responsibility for their schoolwork and other obligations. You can only imagine my surprise when at 11, Andrew reminded me, "Mom, my schoolwork is my responsibility. If I screw up, I'll be the one to suffer and I'll have only myself to blame." (I was thrilled that some of the concepts we were trying to teach were starting to sink in.)

114. Give kids opportunities to solve their own problems.

Dave and I feel that knowing how to manage interpersonal relationships is a skill that needs lots of practice and the earlier kids begin solving their own problems the better. We refused (sometimes this was difficult for us) to take on their problems as our own. We talked and role-played how to deal with an angry friend or a difficult teacher. But we didn't take matters into our hands. We wanted the kids to stand up (respectfully) for themselves and begin to operate in the real world.

115. A strong-willed child will wear you down and will be a step ahead of you every single time. Consider yourself lucky if you catch them "bending the rules."

When Jamie was 12, her friends were the center of her life, but the phone was off limits after 10 p.m. However, to circumvent the rule, she would call the weather, wait for her friend's "call waiting" beep, and click over to her friend. When we found out what she was doing, the phone was removed from her room for 2 weeks.

Another teachable moment occurred when Jamie was at a sleepover with a bunch of girls. In the middle of the night, while the parents were asleep, they snuck out of the house. Thankfully, a neighbor saw the girls, confronted them, and then told the parents. That episode was ripe for discussion.

116. Use a little humor; it helps.

Nagging was a waste of my time and energy so I tried to use humor whenever I could. For example: Taking showers was an issue for Andrew, so I told him I'd know when he started liking girls because he'd begin to shower regularly, but if he started showering now, I'd never know.

117. Kids misbehaving in school? Just tell your kids that you'll come observe them in class. Watch how quickly the questionable behavior disappears!

The Teen Years (14–19)

Sadly, I was very severely disabled by Jamie and Andrew's teenage years and needed help with EVERYTHING. My husband, Dave; family members; friends; neighbors; and paid helpers provided much of the help I needed, but there were many times when the kids, of necessity, had to help me in and out of bed, adjust my position in my scooter, help me in the bathroom, drive me to medical appointments, and much, much more.

As a mom, I knew that teenagers are generally self-centered. It was (and still is) normal for Jamie and Andrew to think of my illness in terms of how it affects them. They were "textbook" teenagers; every day presented new parenting challenges and quick thinking on my part (which is not always possible when you're ill.)

118. Give kids opportunities to "figure it out" without your involvement.

I didn't have the mental energy to get into heated arguments no matter what time of day it was. My response to problems like sharing the car, using the telephone, or scheduling time on the computer was, "I'm not getting involved. You guys work it out." Jamie and Andrew learned to resolve conflicts and became excellent negotiators and communicators.

The kids constantly tested the limits and pushed for independence. Sometimes I felt like I was back to those "terrible twos" again, only now they "had attitude" and could argue and debate. As 16-year-old Jamie told me, "You have to let me grow up and try new things. It's the only way I'll learn."

119. Present opportunities for negotiations and compromise.

I also tried to phrase my questions in a way that gave the kids some options/control in their lives and took their schedules into consideration. For example, "When would you be available for 2 hours to pack up and deliver the books we want to donate to the library?" We'd negotiate and compromise in an effort to seek a solution we could all live with.

120. Curfews! This was a topic ripe for discussion because the kids wanted more control and there was always a friend or two whose parents were more liberal than we were.

When the kids were about 16, we began asking them, "What time do you think you'll be home?" When they balked at our "need to know," we offered this explanation. "It would give us an idea when to expect you and if you didn't show up, we'd know that you might need help and we could begin looking for you." If they knew they were going to be delayed, they needed to call us.

Because I was unable to get out of bed myself to check to see whether they were home, we'd leave the hall light on. When they got home, they'd turn out the light.

121. Teenagers need their space and privacy; it's a natural part of growing up.

Just as I needed space from them, I tried hard to give them space, too. Asking them questions like, "What's wrong?" "What happened?" "What's bothering you?" were not helpful. And it was never easy to have to wait until they were ready, if ever, to share what was going on in their lives.

I wanted to respect their need for privacy, so I tried to be ready to listen when they wanted to talk. My perceptive and direct daughter, Jamie, once told me, "Mom I just want you to listen. I don't want you to tell me what to do." It's important for teenagers to know that you "hear them."

I'm still learning how to listen when the kids just want to vent, and I share my opinions sparingly. Otherwise, I'm likely to cut the conversation short. Comments like, "That's got to be hard . . . I'm sorry this has been so frustrating for you. I know you'll tell me if there is something you want me to do. I know it's disappointing that there are no easy answers . . ." keep the lines of communication open.

122. Parents must have interests and activities of their own.

One day when I must have asked too many questions, Andrew told me that I "had to get a life" of my own. He was right! So I began focusing on doing more things that I enjoyed like writing, reading, and spending time with my friends. It allowed me to take a step back and create more space for the kids to grow.

123. Even though your kids may look like adults, they aren't. Be sure to give them hugs and tell them you love them.

Final Thoughts . . .

Over the years, there were many, many times I worried about my worth as a mother. I felt my kids did more for me than I did for them. I felt that my presence in their lives was a burden and perhaps their lives would be easier if I weren't here. However, when Jamie was 25, she went through a rough time when her "perfect" life seemed to be falling apart. We talked nightly on the phone. As mature and self-sufficient as she was, she still needed me to be her sounding board, cheerleader, confidant, and friend. After every phone call, I thanked God I was still here for her.

Several months later, Jamie and I had lunch. After lunch, we stopped in the restroom. As my beautiful daughter looked in the mirror, I caught her looking at my reflection. Quietly, as though giving voice to sacred thoughts, she said, "I can't imagine how I would have gotten through the last few months without you. Aren't you happy that you're still here?" Yes, Jamie, I am!

Even though we may not be the active, energetic, and healthy parents we would like to be, we have to remember our irreplaceable role in our kids' lives. No matter what our challenges are, we have a responsibility to our children to love, guide, and provide a safe and stable place for them. If or when that becomes difficult, we must use all the resources at our disposal to create a healthy environment for them.

CHAPTER 9

Your House and Home

I spend a great deal of time in my home, so I have tried to create an environment where I can be safe, independent, and productive. In 1999, my husband, Dave, and I built an accessible, custom home. It has barrier-free entrances, widened doorways, grab bars in the bathroom, lowered light switches, and raised electrical outlets. However, before we built this house, we did two major remodeling projects to our old house to make it more accessible. In many cases, we found that the most valuable accessibility improvements generally cost less than $50 to $100. These products are easy to install or are do-it-yourself projects.

Two of my favorite and most inexpensive products that help me all around the house are:

1. Rubber bands: I wind them around kitchen tools, bottles, cleaning-product spray cans, my handheld shower handle, and other household objects to improve my ability to grasp and hold on to items.

2. Rubberized (waffle weave) squares or shelf liner: I use the squares to open jars and bottles and keep small items from sliding or moving around on the table or countertop. When I use the shelf liner as a place mat, my dishes don't slide around. Used under a mixing bowl, the bowl stays in one place. You'll find this product in the kitchen section of discount department stores.

Getting Started—Making Your Home More Accessible

3. If you could benefit from a more accessible home environment, but you don't know where to start, contact your local Independent Living Center (ILC), Aging and Disability Resource Center (ADRC), or Aging-in-Place agency. They will direct you to reputable professionals to evaluate your needs, help you find a Certified Environmental Access Consultant (CEAC) or an Aging-in-Place Specialist (CAPS), and funding sources you may want to contact. CEAC or CAPS are builders and remodelers highly trained in accessibility standards and solutions. Before hiring any contractor, ask to speak with satisfied customers.

4. If you rent rather than own, the Americans with Disabilities Act requires landlords to make "reasonable accommodations" for people with disabilities. However, it is up to the landlord to determine what is reasonable, something the landlord usually decides based on cost and how universal any changes might be for future tenants. If you need grab bars installed in the bathroom, offset hinges installed, or a different type of doorknob, ask your landlord to provide these changes. More extensive changes may be allowed if you or a service agency provides all or part of the funding.

5. Smart-home technology can make your whole house more accessible than ever before with the touch of a finger. From any location with access on a smartphone, tablet, or computer, you are able to control your lights, temperature, TVs, appliances, security cameras, and more. Search online for "home automation products and systems" or "smart-home technology."

Home Accessibility

Lighting and Light Switches

6. Replace traditional light switches with rocker panel or pressure-sensitive switches. Available in lighted or unlighted versions, they

can be turned on and off by pressing with an arm, elbow, or palm of the hand, requiring less fine motor control.

7. A dimmer switch allows you to adjust lights in a room so that one person may work or read without disturbing others.

8. Wall-switch extenders lower a light switch 13 to 15 inches below the actual switch; this makes it easier to turn on and off from wheelchair height. Some extenders mount over a standard single light switch; others replace the existing wall plate using the same screws. These devices are easy to attach and will not scratch or damage walls.

9. Install a lamp converter that fits into the socket and bypasses the on–off switch, making any metal base lamp "touch-sensitive." When you screw in a three-way light bulb, the light gets brighter with each successive touch and then finally turns off.

10. Replace your current lamp(s) with touch-sensitive lamps. These are readily available at home and discount stores.

11. Light-emitting diode (LED) touch pads connected to a lamp require very little pressure to turn lights on and off.

12. Motion-detecting lights and night-lights are readily available to make nighttime movement safer inside or outside your home.

Doorknobs, Doors, and Doorways

13. Replace regular doorknobs with lever handles, or purchase a rubber lever that fits over any standard doorknob. Lever handles are easy to operate—just push down with your hand, arm, or elbow. Lever handles are available at most home-improvement stores.

14. If you use a wheelchair in the house, install U-shaped handles on every doorway. Use them to help pull yourself through the doorway.

15. If the bathroom doorway is too narrow to accommodate a scooter or wheelchair, remove the door. Replace it with a tension rod and an opaque (or black) shower curtain for privacy. Hanging a couple of colorful beach towels is another inexpensive solution for a temporary mobility challenge.

16. To widen doorways by ½ to ¾ inch, carefully pry off the door jamb strips on one or both sides of the door.

17. Install offset hinges that allow the door to swing out and away from the doorway, increasing the door opening by 2 to 3 inches. You can find offset hinges in your local home-building-supply store and online.

18. Keep door hinges well oiled.

19. If a door scrapes along a rug, plane the bottom to make it open and close more easily.

To plane the bottom of a door, without the bother of removing it, put a large piece of coarse sandpaper on the floor under the door (padding it with newspaper if necessary to create a good contact surface) and then move the door back and forth a few times until it swings easily.

20. To make it easier to close a door behind you, tie a 24"-long rope or cord around the doorknob and let it hang down. As you walk through the door, grab the rope and pull the door shut behind you.

21. Attach one cup hook to the door near the knob and a second cup hook to the door jamb on the hinge side. Tie a string or chain between the hooks, and pull it as you go through the doorway. The door will close behind you.

22. Attach spring closures, like those on an old-fashioned screen door.

23. Protect your doors from wheelchair scratches by installing a clear plastic, chrome, or brass kick plate at their base. These are available wherever building supplies are sold or through home-decorating catalogs.

Under Lock and Key

24. Someone who uses a wheelchair or scooter may not be able to get to the door before a visitor or delivery person leaves. To solve this problem, have a qualified electrician install a doorbell or intercom communication system. The system works like this: When a visitor rings the doorbell, every telephone in the house starts to ring. When you answer the telephone, it works like an intercom so that you can communicate with the person waiting outside. If you are on the phone when a visitor arrives, a call-waiting tone will sound to alert you.

25. Some door-answering systems allow you to unlock the door from your telephone. However, these systems only work with hard-wired, landline phones, not cellular phones.

26. A wireless, remote-door-entry system allows access to your home without traditional keys. A battery-powered key fob, similar to those used in automobiles, remotely activates your door lock from over 150 feet away, even while the user remains seated or in bed. The device is mounted to any wooden door, operates cylinder and night-latch (deadbolt) locks, and can be used in conjunction with traditional key locks. For maximum security, the easy-to-program and reprogram fobs use a "rolling code" that changes each time the door is released. Consult a locksmith or security specialist for details.

27. Admit visitors without having to unlock or open your exterior door by keeping a garage door opener in the house. When you want to let someone in, press the garage door opener from inside the house, and let your guest in through the garage entrance.

28. Adaptive key devices fit on your regular key and give better leverage to make holding and turning keys easier. Hardware stores and home-health-care stores have different styles from which to choose. Be sure to try them first to see which works best for you.

Ramps, Railings, Stairs, and Support Poles

29. Plan building a ramp to your home carefully; it may not be as easy as you think.

> *When we needed wheelchair access to our (old) house, Dave and I realized that our front door provided the easiest place to add a ramp. So, one day Dave and his buddy decided they would take on the project. They spent the day measuring, planning, designing, purchasing the supplies, and constructing the ramp. At the end of the day, they wanted me to try it. The minute I opened the front door, I realized there was a BIG problem. The ramp started at the threshold of the open door and went down. There was no landing on which I could start my descent. And getting back into the house was impossible because I couldn't hold the scooter steady while trying to open the door. We needed a platform on the top of the ramp. Back to the drawing board . . . .*

30. If a door is at the top or bottom of the ramp, there should be a level area in front of the door; a platform 5-feet wide by 3-feet long is recommended to enable a person in a wheelchair to unlock and open the door.

31. Whenever possible, put railings on both sides of a ramp. Railing height above ramps is a matter of personal preference. The average-sized person usually finds that a height of 35 to 36 inches works well; if you are short, you may want to consider a railing 32 to 34 inches high.

32. The railing itself should be 1¼ to 1½ inches in diameter and provide a 1½-inch clearance from any obstruction, such as a wall.

33. If your doorway threshold is less than 3 inches, create an easy low-cost "ramp" by using a flexible, vinyl, antiskid surface floor mat like you would use under a desk chair. Depending on the height of the threshold, you may need to support the mat by placing a board or book(s) under the mat inside the house and outside the entrance. Floor mats are sold at office-supply stores.

34. Aluminum ramps are economical and easy to install. Because every situation is different, consult with accessibility experts who can help you decide what type of ramp design is best for you.

35. Consider purchasing a portable ramp. For an idea of what is available, as well as tools for choosing and calculating the right ramp, visit www.discountramps.com.

36. If you don't have room for a ramp or your home design makes it impossible, consider putting in a lift. Lifts can help you get up a few steps in the garage or from one floor to another and are less expensive than elevators.

37. If you need a little assistance getting up or down a step or two, consider installing the Flip-A-Grip Doorway Assist Handle. It mounts in the doorway and folds out of the way so it does not block access when not in use. It glows in the dark so it is easy to find in low- or no- light situations. They are sold online and at discount department stores.

38. Install hand railings on both sides of a stairway so that you have support going up and down stairs.

39. Basement stairs will be safer if you add abrasive rubber treads to each step. For added safety, paint the edge of the steps with luminous paint to make them more visible. To improve the lighting in the stairwell, use at least a 100-watt bulb.

40. Save steps and attract the attention of someone who is upstairs/ downstairs by turning the light switch on and off a few times. The flashing lights will get the person's attention even if the volume on the TV or stereo is cranked up.

41. Install a floor-to-ceiling pole, such as the Guardian Safe-T-Pole™, by the bed, toilet, living-room chair, and dining-room table;

use them as a steadying or balancing aid or to help you get to a standing position. The attractive, durable, heavy-gauge steel poles are held in place by controlled tension, requiring no special tools or structural changes for installation. These are sold online and at discount department stores.

42. The SuperPole™ system is a modular support system that provides assistance with standing, transferring, or moving in bed. The floor-to-ceiling pole is installed by simple jackscrew expansion.

43. Advantage Rail™ is a floor-mounted support rail that promotes safe and independent standing and transfers. The horizontal rail pivots to move with you in safe, small steps, yet locks in place in an instant in case of a loss of balance, need for rest, or to assist you to a seated position. It's also available in a portable model that quickly secures and releases from a low-profile floor-mounted plate, so that you can take it with you when traveling or simply move out of the way when not needed. Additional floor plates can be purchased to use the portable Advantage Rail in multiple locations.

Faucets and Sinks

44. If your faucet has separate controls for hot and cold water, consider installing wrist blades. Wrist blades are wide, wing-type handles that are operated by pushing with the forearm, wrist, or heel of the hand. They are available at most plumbing-supply stores and hardware stores.

45. Kitchen faucets are generally longer than bathroom faucets.

When it became too difficult for me to stretch my arms out to reach the bathroom faucet, we replaced it with a kitchen faucet. It made all the difference!

46. Touch-free or touch-sensitive faucets are readily available at home-improvement stores and where plumbing supplies are sold. They come in a variety of styles to fit any home décor.

Furniture and Rugs

47. Place a clear plastic or vinyl chair protector on your upholstered dining-room chairs and gain several advantages—it prevents spills from staining fabric and makes it easier to change position or slide on and off the chair seat.

48. Use sturdy and stable furniture. Generally, the best type of chair has a relatively straight back, a firm shallow seat, and armrests for added support. Avoid low, overstuffed sofas and chairs that make sitting and standing more difficult.

49. To make it easier to get up from a chair or sofa, furniture should be approximately 17 inches off the ground.

50. Adjust the height of your furniture by adding or removing casters or putting measured blocks of wood under each leg until you have the desired height.

51. It is easier to get out of a chair by scooting forward to the edge of the seat, spreading your feet apart, and rocking back and forth to build up momentum.

52. Remove throw rugs. Walking or wheeling on vinyl, ceramic, or wood floors is easier than walking or wheeling on thick carpet. (Use caution: Vinyl, ceramic, or wood floors may be slippery when wet.)

53. To make walking on carpet easier, choose a flat, tightly woven or loop style, not a plush or sculptured style. A high-density or commercial pad under the carpet will last longer and creates a more stable walking surface.

The Bathroom

Organizing the Bathroom

54. Keep everything you need within easy reach. Store cotton swabs, dental floss swords, supplements, and so on in clear containers so you can see at a glance what's inside.

55. Use a toothbrush holder to hold an assortment of makeup brushes, nail-care products, and/or a spoon for taking liquid medication.

56. Use a spice rack placed at eye level to hold medications or small items that might easily be "lost" in a drawer.

57. Keep your jewelry organized and easy to find.

I use ice cube trays to hold my earrings; the little cups keep earrings from getting jumbled and they are easy to see and retrieve.

58. Create your own drawer organizers to fit your needs.

I made my own drawer organizers using binder clips and large paperclips to join boxes, baskets, and plastic containers together. It's easy to reorganize drawers to fit changing needs.

59. Turntables on the counter or in bathroom closets make items easy to retrieve.

60. Reserve a drawer in the bathroom for clean undergarments. That way, when you have finished showering, you have everything you need to start getting dressed.

61. Place mirrors where you need them. The medicine-chest mirror may be too high for children or people who sit in a wheelchair. Purchase a telescoping mirror that either clamps to the sidewall of the vanity or sits on top of the vanity counter. Telescoping mirrors feature adjustable, swivel-type necks that you can move to various positions.

62. Magnifying mirrors have a regular mirror on one side and the other side magnifies, making it perfect for makeup application or shaving. Some styles hang around your neck, leaving your hands free.

63. Substitute a wash mitt or soft sponge for the usual washcloth. Sponges are easier to use if your hands are weak.

64. Pop-up tissues and wipes are easier to grab than the kind that lie flat in the box.

65. Install a touch-free soap dispenser or use a liquid soap pump dispenser.

66. Transfer hair care products, body spray, and water from difficult-to-use pump applicators to decorative trigger-handle spray bottles found at drug, kitchen, and bath stores.

The Toilet

67. If you find that the height of standard toilet seats makes it difficult to get on and off the toilet, install a wall-mounted toilet seat at a level that is convenient for you.

68. Add an adjustable, portable toilet seat that will increase the height 4 to 7 inches. Some models provide armrests for added support. Portable seats are easy to attach to any toilet; to safely use bathrooms away from home, purchase a tote bag so that you can take the seat with you.

To make it easier for me and the person helping me, I keep a portable toilet seat at my son's, daughter's, and mother's house for when we visit. When we travel by car elsewhere, we take one with us.

69. A self-powered, lifting commode chair helps users sit and rise with less effort. Lifting most of a user's weight, it provides safe, controlled support while sitting and standing. Look for a commode chair that has a removable catch basin so that it can stand alone in a bedroom or be used over a standard toilet.

70. If flushing a standard toilet is difficult, try adding an extra-large flush handle or a foot-flusher attachment.

71. If wiping yourself is difficult, a bidet attachment will wash you and no wiping is necessary. Many models are available, so check your options online.

The Tub and Shower

72. Purchase a shower chair or bench so you can sit while you shower. There are dozens of styles and sizes to choose from, so choose one that provides the support you need.

73. If getting into or out of the bathtub to take a shower is difficult for you, purchase a bath and shower chair that has an overhanging bench. Two legs of this device stand in the tub and two legs stand on the bathroom floor. You sit on the bench with your legs on the outside of the tub. Then you lift one leg at a time into the tub. Once your legs are in the tub, you slide your bottom over and sit as you would in a chair. To make sliding over on the bench easier, sprinkle powder or cornstarch on the surface. To determine what kind of chair/bench would work best for you, visit a home-health or medical-supply store in your community.

74. Consider installing a walk-in tub or one of the many styles of bathtub assists that lower you safely into the bath, and smoothly raise you up again. Visit a bathroom-design shop, home-improvement or home-health store, or do a search online for styles that are available.

75. Consider putting the items you use in the tub and shower in a shower caddy to keep products off the floor.

76. Use decorative nonslip tape or decals in the tub or shower for improved traction.

77. If you use a rubber mat, periodically toss it in the washing machine with soap and a little bleach to remove that slippery soap-film buildup.

Grab Bars

78. Never grab onto towel racks or soap dish holders for support. Grab bars must be securely anchored to wall studs; hire a professional to do the installation.

79. Before installing grab bars, determine where they would provide the most help. A space the width of a clenched fist (about 1½ inches) should exist between the grab bar and the wall.

80. Vinyl-covered grab rails are easier to grip and absorb less heat than metal.

The Bedroom

81. To improve your comfort in bed when you have a chronic or painful condition, you need a comfortable mattress. No one but you can determine what is best for you. Whether you choose a traditional innerspring, a memory foam, an adjustable Sleep Number® bed, a waterbed, or an organic cotton or hypoallergenic mattress, do your research first. Compare and read reviews of different kinds of mattresses. When you're ready to buy, ask about a 30-day sleep guarantee, which ensures the company will take the mattress back and return your old one if the new one doesn't work for you.

82. Natural organic wool provides warmth and cushioning when in bed.

83. Organic wool batten mattresses, mattress toppers, bedding, and pillows are chemical free, hypoallergenic, and naturally fire resistant. Their natural fiber cools in the summer and warms in the winter.

84. When you make the bed, minimize the amount of walking involved by making up one side of a bed completely, and then finish the other side.

85. Use a 2-foot stick or dowel, with a plastic-coated cup hook attached to one end, to help you arrange the blanket and sheet when you get in or out of bed. The hook allows you to arrange the bed coverings easily; however, it cannot be used with an open-weave or thermal blanket, because the hook snags the threads.

86. Choose bed covers that provide warmth without weight.

87. Woven-knit sheets are easy to put on the mattress because the corners stretch easily, but, if turning over in bed is difficult, woven-satin sheets will help you slide more easily. You can also turn over more easily if you wear nylon or silk pajamas.

I don't recommend that you sleep on satin sheets while wearing nylon or silk pajamas—the combination might be so slippery that you could slip out of bed.

88. If turning over or changing sleeping positions in bed is difficult, consider pushing the side of the bed up against the bedroom wall and installing a railing or grab bar. Anchor the railing to a stud and install it at a height that makes turning easier.

89. The Smart-Rail™ is an innovative bed-assist rail designed for those requiring a little help for moving, standing, and/or transferring in and out of bed. Unlike fixed-style bed rails, Smart-Rail can unlock and pivot outward to provide better standing support with less reaching and twisting.

90. Install wall-mounted, swing-arm lamps on either side of the bed. This frees up space on the nightstand for other items and you can move the light where you need it.

91. If you have trouble sitting or standing when getting out of bed, the Bedside Assistant® may provide the support you need. This adjustable device slips under either side of a standard mattress and gives the user sturdy handles to grab onto when rolling over, repositioning, or pulling to an upright position (www .BedHandles.com).

92. Keep a flashlight by the entrance to your bedroom. Use it at night when you have turned off the light and need to illuminate the path to your bed. Then keep the flashlight on your nightstand, so that it will be handy if you need to get out of bed in the middle of the night. If you have a smartphone, you can use its flashlight mode.

93. Organize your bedroom closets for easy access by making shelves and clothing rods low enough to reach without straining.

94. If you have vision problems, mobility issues, or someone else assists you with dressing, consider organizing your closet by hanging everything you need for one outfit (skirt, blouse, sweater, scarf, belt, even jewelry) on one hanger. That way you have everything you need in one place.

Housecleaning and Chores

95. Use a child-sized broom or adaptive equipment, such as extended handles for dusters or brushes; this will allow you to sweep the kitchen floor while sitting.

96. If you need additional support when raking, sweeping, or handling any kind of long-handled implement, the Robohandle®, with its pistol grip and arm support, may make your work easier. This device can also be added to a cane or crutches to improve support (www.robohandle.com).

97. A simple fix for dusting hard-to-reach places is to use rubber bands to attach a sock to a yardstick.

98. Make quick work of wiping up crumbs on the floor by sweeping them into a pile; then wet a paper towel, wring it out, and use it to wipe up the crumbs. This technique works well, especially if you can't coordinate the use of a dustpan and broom.

99. Conserve energy by storing mops, brooms, and other housecleaning tools in gravity or friction tool holders that mount on your wall or door. Some models are screw mounted; others are adhesive backed to make installation easier, especially for people who have difficulty managing heavy drills or screwdrivers. Once installed, you may hang items simply by inserting the handle through the bottom of a rubberized center core that grabs the tool handle and holds it firmly until you lift and release it.

100. Collect clothes in one place and transfer them to the laundry area in a wheeled cart, if possible. When the laundry is dry, put it back into the cart, wheel it into the family room, and teach the children how to fold their laundry and then put it away. Make the chore more enjoyable by listening to music, a radio, or watching a favorite TV show as they fold.

101. Have family members help with the laundry by posting an index card near the washer and dryer indicating how much and what kind of cleaning products to use, water levels, and temperature settings for each type of clothing. Remind them to keep Velcro® fasteners closed so that the garment does not collect lint or snag other garments.

102. If the laundry area is in the basement, plan to remain there until the laundry is done. Create a place to relax while waiting, stocked with a phone, books, magazines, crafts, or work projects to occupy you while you wait. Hang clothes promptly after they dry to minimize the need for ironing. Sit down when you iron to save energy.

Home Safety

When living with multiple sclerosis, it's especially important that we prepare for emergencies and unexpected or natural disasters. Here are items you may want to consider to increase your safety and reduce your stress.

103. Before an emergency occurs, get family members and caregivers together to agree on the following: exit routes from your home; a local meeting place outside your home; a person to contact outside your region who, when local phone systems are overloaded, can relay information to family or friends across the country.

104. Plan ahead for power outages. People who use power-dependent equipment, such as oxygen, environmental control units, electric beds and lifts, and so forth, should notify their local utility company so that everyone is prepared should an emergency power outage occur. (Your doctor will need to fill out a form indicating your medical problem and the type of equipment you use.) In an emergency, the utility company will make every attempt to restore service to your location as soon as possible. However, it still is your responsibility to have a backup power source.

105. Notify your local utilities of your special needs and equipment and ask them to alert you when repairs, meter changes, or routine maintenance necessitate that the power is turned off. It will give you time to make backup arrangements.

106. Make sure everyone in the house, including children, knows where the main water shut-off valve is located and how and when to use it, especially if you are not able to get downstairs yourself. Keep the valve in good working order by turning it off and on every 6 months.

107. Let your local fire department know if you might have difficulty escaping from your home in the event of a fire. They will keep this information on file.

108. Show your children how the smoke detectors work, what they sound like, and what they should do when they hear one go off. Be sure to discuss how important it might be to run to a neighbor's house to get help and call the fire department, emphasizing that leaving the house to get help would not mean they are abandoning their pets or family members. Contact your local fire department for more information on teaching home fire safety.

109. Install smoke alarms in every sleeping room and outside any sleeping areas. Keep smoke out of the bedroom by sleeping with your door closed. It will give you precious moments to escape.

110. If anyone in your household is deaf or if your own hearing is diminished, consider installing a smoke alarm that uses a flashing light or vibration to alert you to a fire emergency.

111. Test all your home smoke alarms twice a year and replace batteries when necessary.

We test ours every spring and fall when the time changes.

112. Keep a fire extinguisher in the kitchen, garage, near a fireplace—anywhere a fire is more likely to break out. When you call 911 for help, tell the dispatcher about any special information they need to know (i.e., the person is a hoarder; is bedridden; has mental health issues; has cognitive, sensory, or mobility impairments; is frail and elderly). This information will help the rescue effort. Be sure to include where the person is located in the building and any special equipment he or she might need.

113. Know where the "spare key" is located (e.g., to the right of the backdoor under the "Believe" paver next to the blue flowerpot), so the 911 operator can relay the information to rescue personnel.

114. If you call for emergency fire, police, or rescue services and the door to your home is locked, emergency personnel will knock down your door to gain access.

115. Put a label with your address and telephone number on your phone or in a prominent place for aides or helpers in your home who may not recall the information in a stressful situation.

116. Always make sure that the numbers on your house are clearly visible from the street. Paint them on a curb with a florescent paint, or on a mailbox, or make sure that a porch light illuminates your address.

117. Wear a medical-alert pendant.

I've worn one for more than 30 years and I wouldn't go a day without it. I've only used it twice, but it saved me great pain and injury both times. When I push the button to activate the service, an operator from the call center calls to find out if I need help. If I don't or am unable to respond, they call my local 911 operator to request that they send help to my home. Check with your doctor, local hospital, or online for more information.

118. Install an electronic driveway sensor. These sensors, mounted beside your driveway, will flash and sound a chime alerting you when a car approaches, giving you extra time to get to the door. For added security or if someone is deaf or hard of hearing, an optional lamp controller will turn on a light or radio in the house. Some devices allow you to set up different functions based on whether a car is arriving or departing.

119. Keep walks, driveways, and ramps free of snow and ice with granular or liquid deicer, available at your local hardware or home-supply store. Some applications may be applied before bad weather is expected and have lasting effects up to 2 weeks.

120. Remove outdoor obstacles like warmer weather planters and decorations.

121. Consider installing solar-powered lighting to light your way when dark nights come early.

122. If your mail is delivered to a mailbox at the curb or at the mouth of your driveway, you may qualify to have your mail delivered directly to your door. Known as a "hardship medical delivery," this service is available by submitting a written request with documentation from your doctor to your local postmaster, who will make the decision about the service.

123. Consider using delivery services for prescription medicines, groceries, stamps, and more. Just ask whether this service is available where you live.

124. Use baby monitors, nanny cams, or Wi-Fi cameras to monitor activities in your home and outside from your computer or smartphone. Many styles are available online or in baby or electronics departments.

Now that you have a few new ideas for making your home more accessible, safer, and easier to take care of, create your own shortcuts, tips, and time-savers. Then use your "free time" to enjoy life with your friends and family.

CHAPTER 10

Mealtime

The kitchen is the busiest room in our house. Ever since my diagnosis, preparing and cooking meals has been a family affair. In those early years, I worked at making the kitchen more efficient and well organized. I continue doing the same today. I hope the tips and ideas here will inspire you to make your life easier in the kitchen.

Making Your Kitchen More Accessible

1. Get rid of clutter and broken or rarely used pots, pans, dishes, and utensils.

2. Rearrange items, putting things close to where they are used.

   I keep silverware near the kitchen table, cookware near the stove, and cleaning supplies near the sink.

   I place frequently used items in the front of the cabinets and drawers and put seldom used items in the back.

   If I use measuring spoons, paring knives, or spatulas in different parts of the kitchen, I purchase duplicates and keep them where they are used.

3. Make deep or difficult-to-reach countertop corners easier to use by blocking off the corner. Then, canisters and small appliances can't be pushed or moved out of reach.

4. Use lazy Susan turntables in kitchen and storage cabinets, the refrigerator, and on counters and tables to bring items within easy reach.

5. Install under-cabinet lights to improve lighting on the counter-tops. Better lighting reduces my fatigue and increases safety.

6. Place heavy or frequently used appliances, such as toasters, blenders, or stand mixers, on a countertop, instead of storing them in a cabinet.

7. If you do not have space to keep appliances on the counter, consider purchasing a mixer/appliance lift that makes it easier to raise and lower the appliance to counter level. Search online for "appliance lifts" and other kitchen counter and cupboard solutions.

When the refrigerator door was too difficult for me to open because the seal was too tight, my husband Dave adjusted the pitch of the refrigerator to make the door open more easily. Unfortunately, that didn't totally solve the problem. So we placed a small piece of masking tape over the magnetic area on the door. The door still closes tightly and thankfully, is now much easier to open.

8. Use electrical appliances rather than manual ones whenever possible, including food processors, mixers, blenders, and can openers.

9. If you have difficulty opening jars and bottles, cordless jar and bottle openers may help. Some models mount under a cabinet within easy reach; simply press the top of the jar into the opener and the power twist cone starts automatically.

10. Wear rubber gloves or use thin, rubberized, waffle-like squares to make opening jars easier.

When vacuum-sealed jars became too difficult for me to open, I asked the clerk at the checkout to "break the seal" and then reclose the jar.

11. Store heavy cans and food items at a height that's easiest for you to manage.

12. Try using a stool with casters that roll to eliminate unnecessary steps.

13. Use a wheeled utility cart to transport numerous and/or heavy items from counter to table or table to sink.

14. Hang utensils on magnetic strips, organizers, pegboard, or under cabinets to provide easier accessibility.

15. Replace your kitchen gadgets and utensils with modern ergonomically designed products. Spoons, peelers, graters, spatulas, scrapers, and so on, all come with large, easy-to-grip, cushioned handles.

16. Save energy and eliminate extra serving pieces by using cookware designed for oven-to-table use.

17. Use an adaptive cutting board that best suits your needs. A cutting board with prongs or spikes will hold items in place as they are being cut. Some have suction cups on the bottom to hold the board in place.

18. A multifunctional tool designed for one-handed use, the Swedish Cutting Board can be used to slice and grate food or hold mixing and salad bowls while stirring. Features include a vise to hold larger items, including jars and mixing bowls; a stainless-steel spike insert that holds vegetables for slicing (insert can be turned over to provide a smooth cutting surface); and rubber suction feet to hold the 12 × 11-inch board securely to a countertop or table.

I use an Alaskan ulu knife to cut and chop everything. The curved blade and the companion cutting-board bowl (flat on the bottom and curved to meet the knife blade on the other), makes one-handed cutting easier (www.theULUfactory.com).

Meal Planning and Preparation

As my disability increased and fatigue drained my energy, I made compromises and changes to the way I got meals on the table. Even today, I use these same tips and strategies.

19. Gather items you need to prepare a meal; then sit while doing the actual food preparation.

20. Purchase foods in a form that requires minimal preparation— dehydrated, frozen, canned, packaged mixes, and so on.

21. Purchase mixed salad greens in a bag, cut and cleaned carrots, cut up fresh fruits and vegetables and more.

When I have ready-to-eat fresh foods available, I make better dietary choices. The foods may be a little more expensive, but I need to eat healthyfully, especially on those days when I'm not feeling well.

22. Prepare a double batch of a recipe and freeze half for later use.

23. Use a microwave oven or slow cooker to cut down on cooking and cleanup time.

24. Instead of trying to put clear plastic wrap tightly around a container you want to put in the microwave, put the food in a cereal bowl and set a saucer on top of the bowl. Or purchase a light-weight cover designed for microwave cooking.

25. Slide heavy items along the countertop rather than lifting them.

26. Line baking pans with foil to minimize cleanup.

27. If baked-on food is too difficult to clean, soak pots and pans in hot water and baking soda and cover; the soda loosens the cooked-on food, often eliminating the need for scrubbing.

28. Wipe off any spills on oven racks as soon as possible; clean oven shelves slide in and out more easily.

29. Bake drop cookies as bar cookies. Spread all the cookie dough on a jelly-roll pan, then bake and cut the baked cookies into squares. (Lower the heat about 50° and cook about 10 minutes longer.)

30. Prepare marinated meats, which are easier to cut and chew.

31. If chewing foods like carrots and other hard vegetables is difficult, chop, steam, stew, or grate them to make them easier to chew without losing their nutritional value.

32. Enlist help in the kitchen. When you involve your children in cooking and other mealtime preparations, remember that things that are obvious to adults may not always be obvious to children. For example, there is a vast difference between sugar and salt, but they both look like tiny white crystals; label the containers so children don't substitute one for the other. Put a dab of red nail polish to mark the off position on stove burner controls, so you can see at a glance, even from across the room, that the burner is off.

33. Be sure to allow extra time when children are helping you cook. Keep the atmosphere light and your sense of humor intact.

34. Promote teamwork at mealtime; give everyone a job to do (fill water glasses, carry hot dishes to the table, open wine bottles, serve coffee, etc.). I ask guests to help clear the table and refrigerate leftovers.

35. Making simple changes in your diet, such as having salad dressing served on the side, eating baked or steamed foods rather than fried foods, eating more fresh fruits and vegetables, and reducing your intake of processed foods, is beneficial for everyone.

Cooking Safety

36. Allow plenty of time for each kitchen task. Don't begin cooking when you're tired or rushed for time. Fatigue or haste might make you stumble, drop a pan, or burn yourself.

37. Always use proper-size pans on burners. Don't put a small pot on a large burner.

38. Turn the handles of pots and pans toward the inside of the stove to avoid accidently bumping them and knocking them off.

39. Never store food, cookware, or small appliances in the oven. You may forget they're in there. Plus, if someone else uses your oven, he or she is not likely to look inside before turning it on.

40. Have cues and reminders to help you remember that you have food cooking on the stove.

I always set a timer (on the stove, my cellphone, or a portable timer), when I have something cooking in the oven or on the stovetop. Then, if I leave the room or get a phone call, I don't forget about the cooking food.

If I'm working in the kitchen and know that I will be leaving the house, I put a potholder on top of my purse to remind me to turn off the stove before I leave.

41. Never reach over a hot burner to remove food.

42. If you have a hood over your stove, you may want to put colorful tape around it to avoid bumping into it.

43. Use mitten-type hot pads to remove food from the stove or oven. They're less likely to slip out of position and provide greater protection than regular potholders. For extra added safety, use mitts with asbestos palms.

44. Extra-long, heat-resistant oven mitts that extend to the elbow protect your forearms from steam burns and from touching the sides of the oven.

45. Never use a towel or wet potholder to remove a hot dish.

46. Keep a lightweight, easy-to-use fire extinguisher in an easy-to-grab place by the stove. Be sure to replace or recharge it regularly.

47. Aluminum cookware, lightweight gadgets, and sharp knives help you conserve energy.

48. Small appliances, like a slow cooker or Crock Pot™, make it easy for you to prepare meals early in the day when energy is usually at its peak. Plus, there's no standing at the stove, no hot pots to handle, and no major mess to clean up at the end of the day.

49. Wear nonflammable materials whenever working in the kitchen. Long-sleeved garments or loose-fitting clothing could get caught in appliances or could catch on fire.

50. If you lack sensation in your hands, keep a floating thermometer in the sink to avoid burns from hot water and wear rubber gloves for added protection.

51. Remove floor rugs, waste cans, and other obstacles that might be in the way.

52. Keep cabinet doors and drawers closed when not in use.

53. Keep knives in a wall-hung knife rack, in a countertop knife holder, or on a magnetic knife rack on the side of a cabinet. The handles are easy to grasp and you're protected from the sharp blades. If you must keep knives in a drawer, put a sheath on them to protect yourself from the blade.

Serving Meals and Cleaning Up

54. You may need to select dinnerware that is easier to manage.

When my hands became too weak to safely handle our dinnerware, we replaced it with Corelle® dishes; they're lightweight and don't break as easily as china. We also replaced heavy pottery mugs with porcelain or china drinking cups.

55. Consider using paper plates to make cleanup easier, especially when you aren't feeling well.

56. Dishes and flatware that contrast with the color of the tabletop will be easier to find for people with vision problems. Some flatware comes with large, easy-to-grip handles in colorful and seasonal designs.

57. Use a dish towel or a hand towel on your lap instead of a napkin; they are bigger, more absorbent, and are less likely to fall on the floor.

58. Cutting pizza into squares makes it easier to handle and eat than cutting it in triangles.

59. Eliminate your sugar bowl and avoid spills by filling a large kitchen salt shaker with sugar. (Be sure to label it.) It's easier to handle and control the flow.

60. Make standing at the sink easier.

Many years ago, when I was having difficulty standing at the kitchen sink to do dishes, I found I could stand better (and longer), if I opened the cabinet door and rested one foot on the floor of the cabinet.

61. Use easy-to-squeeze clips to close bags of partially used foods like pretzels, bread, chips, and so on.

62. When unloading the dishwasher, set the table with the dishes and silverware you will need for the next meal.

Streamlining Grocery Shopping

63. Plan menus for the week before going to the store, and take a shopping list with you.

64. Consider creating two grocery lists—one for high-priority items and the other for nonessentials or items that might wait. Then, if you're suddenly overcome with fatigue, you can easily cut your trip short.

65. Group foods on your list (deli, meat, produce, frozen foods, etc.) to eliminate backtracking. If you create a master grocery list of products you normally shop for and organize it to match the store's layout, you can save time and energy and simply check off the specific items you need.

66. Shop early in the day when you are more rested. Most grocery stores are not as busy first thing in the morning and it is much more relaxing to shop in a store that's not crowded.

67. Call the store to ask when they receive fresh produce, and so on, and when the shelves are fully stocked.

68. For easier shopping, use the same grocery store and learn where various items are located.

I learned in the early years of my diagnosis to choose my grocery store carefully. Even before leaving the house, I mentally ran through a checklist. Where was the handicapped parking located? How safe and maintained was the parking lot? And how many handicapped spaces were there? I thought about the restrooms and their accessibility, how wide the aisles were, how loud the music was, and did the store have adequate lighting? Any one of these "brick and mortar" items could defeat me.

69. When entering a new store, ask for a layout or map of the store so you can save steps and visit only the departments you need to.

70. Use a shopping cart or walker when you shop.

When I was still ambulatory, but beginning to be unsteady on my feet, a grocery cart provided needed stability and made shopping easier and safer.

71. Many grocery stores now have battery-operated carts to make "walking the aisles" easier. They are there for the convenience of their customers who tire easily so do not be embarrassed to use them.

72. If you need assistance reaching items on a shelf, ask a nearby shopper or a sales person for help; if you ask, some stores will have an employee accompany you as you shop.

73. Contact the store manager or owner to arrange for any special services you might need and the best time to receive those services.

74. Take along a magnifying glass on a cord or chain around your neck so you can read the small print on product labels and compare ingredients.

75. If an item at the meat or produce counter is too large to handle, ask the person behind the counter to divide and repackage it into smaller, more manageable portions. Time permitting, butchers will separate ribs, slice a brisket, or butterfly meat if asked.

76. Stock up on paper products, boxed or canned goods, flour, sugar, and things you use regularly, so if the weather keeps you from getting out, you will have the essentials.

77. Ask the bagger not to fill your bags too full. Spread out the items into more bags that will weigh less.

78. Ask that all frozen or perishable foods be put into one bag. Then, when you arrive home, you only need to empty one bag immediately; the other groceries can wait.

79. Some stores offer home delivery, which is especially helpful if you cannot drive or the weather is too hot or cold to venture out.

80. Sometimes stores you shop at regularly may agree to select a few groceries for you and have them ready for you or a neighbor to pick up. Ask store personnel what time of the day would be most convenient for you to pick up your order. If you are unable to leave your car, tell them that you will call when you are in the parking lot.

81. If you want or need special services, avoid shopping on weekends, just before a holiday, or on double-coupon days when the store will likely be busier and more crowded.

82. Check out local shopping and Internet grocery services.

83. Your local social services agency, United Way (dial 211), or Aging and Disability Resource Center can provide information on assistance with transportation, helping hands, and other services to help you with your grocery shopping.

84. Make it easier for someone to grocery shop for you by giving them specific instructions.

When I was no longer able to drive or grocery shop, Dave took over. However, he had these two requests: (a) he wanted a list of what we needed (size, quantity, and brand) and (b) he only wanted to go to the store once a week.

Easier Eating and Drinking

85. Purchase stainless-steel flatware with big bamboo or plastic handles that are easier to grip.

86. Use serrated steak knives for cutting all foods at mealtime.

87. A small salad fork is lighter and easier to handle than a dinner fork.

88. When eating, you'll have better control if you hold the utensil as close as possible to the tines of the fork or the bowl of the spoon.

89. If you have hand tremors, limited coordination, or upper extremity weakness, a swivel utensil, designed for people with tremors, will make it easier to get food to your mouth without spilling. These utensils swivel to maintain a horizontal position even with a 30° tilt of the wrist. Utensils with weighted handles may also help calm tremors.

90. Place two tight rubber bands an inch or so apart around a drinking glass; this will make it easier to grasp and hold onto.

91. Thermal mugs and children's mugs with large handles are easier to grasp than regular glasses or cups.

92. Use insulated mugs and glasses to keep drinks hot or cold without affecting the outside temperature of the glass; this is particularly helpful for people who have lost sensation in their hands or have problems with coordination.

93. The Nosey Cup has an opening for the nose that allows drinking without tilting the head.

94. The Transparent Mug with Drinking Spout has two handles for easy gripping and makes it easier to see the level of the liquid inside. Its wide base prevents tipping.

95. The Kennedy Cup is designed to be used with a straw. Made of dishwasher-safe plastic, its unique design and secure cover make it virtually spill proof.

96. Cups with handles and thumb rests on each side make handling beverages easier. The Artho® Thumbs-Up™ cup is made of plastic, and even though it's insulated, it weighs only 4 ounces.

97. If you need longer straws than those commercially available, purchase some clear tubing at a hardware store and create the length that you need.

98. Baby plates that hold hot water help keep food warm for people who are slow in feeding themselves. The Keep-Warm Dish, made of dishwasher-safe plastic, comes in an adult size. It uses no cords or electricity; just fill with hot water.

99. If you have trouble keeping food from sliding off the plate, try using a glass or metal pie pan instead of a regular plate.

100. To help stabilize a plate, use rubber circles designed to hold soap on the shower wall. The suction cups on one side go on the bottom of the plate while the other side secures the plate to the table.

101. The Inner-Lip™ scooper bowl or plate reduces spills when eating. These dishwasher- and microwave-safe plates and bowls have a nonskid pad on the underside rim that keeps them from moving around and a lip around the edge that keeps food from sliding off.

102. To get a wheelchair close enough to the dinner table to comfortably eat a meal, place a jelly-roll pan (a cookie sheet with sides) or a cafeteria tray lengthwise across the armrests. (If these are not wide enough to rest across the armrests of your wheelchair, have someone cut a board that is the appropriate dimensions for your needs.) Then push the wheelchair close to the table and adjust the edge of your tray to rest flush with the edge of the table. Put your plate and drink on your new custom place mat.

103. You can make eating easier if you elevate your plate. Experiment with different heights. Use a wicker breadbasket, a book, or a sturdy cardboard box to raise the plate to the right level. Once determined, create a more permanent base for eating.

Entertaining

As my multiple sclerosis progressed, we had to change the way we entertained if we wanted to continue to have friends and relatives over to our house for meals. I had to give myself permission to simplify and streamline everything. Use the tips below to help you continue "breaking bread" with family and friends.

104. Prepare and freeze dishes in advance so you only have to thaw or reheat them on the day of the gathering.

105. Serve make-it-yourself meals, like pizza, tacos, or salads, or keep it really simple and just serve wine, cheese, and fruit.

106. Hire a high-school or college student to help serve and clean up.

107. For very special occasions, hire a caterer; they are not as expensive as you might think and save you hours of preparation and cleanup.

108. When we invite friends over for brunch or dinner, they participate in all the activities.

When guests ask, "What can I bring?" I take them up on their offer. I tell them what we need, and let them choose what to bring. Guests know our situation and are happy to bring part of the meal. Visiting friends and relatives also take an active part in helping to get the food on the table and in cleaning up. They are always happy to help. Talking, laughing, and sharing time in the kitchen are all part of the experience when you come to the Schwarz house for a meal.

109. Stay as active and engaged as possible. Your efforts are appreciated.

Now that the children are married and have families of their own, Dave and I continue to work in the kitchen together. Dave cooks the meals but he likes me to be in the kitchen keeping him company and doing what I can—like setting the table, filling water glasses, and getting things out of the refrigerator.

I encourage you to use these tips and ideas to save time and energy, stay safe, and be more efficient in the kitchen. You will have more time to relax and enjoy an extra cup of coffee or your dinner with friends.

CHAPTER 11

Dressing—Looking Your Best

The way I look and dress always has been important to me. After my multiple sclerosis diagnosis, however, I didn't have the strength or energy I needed to get ready for the day like I used to. That meant that I had to find new ways of doing everything from grooming and getting dressed to shopping for clothes and making changes to the type of clothing I wore. It was a slow process. Some things I learned through trial and error, some I learned from professionals (occupational and physical therapists and health aides), and still more I learned from others living with chronic illnesses and conditions. Develop your own tips and strategies for streamlining and getting ready for your day and then "make it a good one."

Grooming

1. To keep your body temperature down, bathing or showering in cool water is recommended for people with MS. Start with warm or tepid water and gradually increase the coolness, giving your body time to adjust.

2. Put on a terry-cloth bathrobe after showering; it makes drying off easier and it feels luxurious.

3. If possible, cut your toenails soon after you bathe; they will be less brittle and easier to cut. A toenail clipper or a pair of scissors with short blades works best. However, if your nails are too

thick, select a heavy-duty pair or consider having them cut by a pedicurist or podiatrist.

4. Purchase combs, hairbrushes, and toothbrushes with large, easy-to-grasp handles.

5. Brushing your teeth twice a day and flossing daily prevents dental problems and diseases. If using a manual toothbrush, dental floss string, and/or flossing "swords" (they look like the letter "C" with floss stretched tight across the opening at the end of a plastic toothpick) are difficult to use because of tremors, weakness, or a lack of fine motor control, consider purchasing an electric toothbrush and water flosser to make brushing and flossing easier. Ask your dentist which style/type may be best for you.

6. If you have difficulty squeezing a toothpaste tube, a toothpaste twister device may make it easier. Some are simple, slotted, key-shaped winders that slide over the end of the toothpaste tube; simply turn to tighten the tube and express the paste.

I use a metal clamp-type clip (similar to a bulldog clip) that I can manage and put it on the bottom of my tube of toothpaste. As I use the toothpaste, I roll up the tube and reposition the clip.

7. If you have difficulty blow-drying your own hair, perhaps because of limited grip or arm strength, consider purchasing a freestanding hand hair dryer holder. With a stable base and moveable neck, you can easily insert the blow dryer handle into the holder at the top and dry your hair, hands-free, simply by turning your head.

Dressing Tips

8. Save time and energy in the morning by laying out your clothing for the next day before you go to bed. This has an added benefit: If you need help with fasteners, buttons, or zippers, you will be able to ask a family member for assistance before he or she leaves for the day.

9. Choose what you wear based on the day's activities. If you plan on swimming, for example, choose an easy-on, easy-off outfit with few buttons, zippers, or ties.

10. If you will be traveling by car, train, or plane, wear an outfit made of a silky or nylon fabric. The slippery fabric makes it much easier to change your position, especially on upholstered seats.

11. If possible, dress once for the day. If you have a meeting or party in the evening, select an outfit that can be dressed up simply. Women can change their whole look by changing jewelry or adding a scarf, sweater, or jacket. Men can put on a tie, vest, sweater, or sport jacket.

12. Always dress a disabled limb first. To undress, take the garment off the good limb first. Unbutton and ease the garment off your shoulders. Reach behind your back and gently tug the garment off.

13. Dress in front of a mirror. This will help you find the sleeves and match up buttons and buttonholes. Button garments from the bottom up, so that you are less likely to skip a button. You might also try buttoning the bottom buttons and then pulling the garment over your head.

14. It's easier to pull slacks up and down if you wear underwear made of nylon instead of cotton.

15. If you are inactive, you will be more likely to feel cold. Dress in layers and you'll have better control over your body temperature as spaces between layers trap warm air. The more loose-fitting the layers the better; this will make it easier to take off or put on a layer as needed to stay comfortable.

16. To tie a necktie using only one hand, take a bulldog clip or a spring-type clothespin and use it to clip the narrow end of the necktie to the front of your buttoned shirt, then tie the tie as usual. Once you have tied your necktie, loosen it just enough so that you can lift it over your head to take it off. The next time you put on

the tie, it will already be tied; you just slide the knot tighter and you're ready to go.

17. To eliminate tying a necktie altogether, wear a clip-on or zipper tie.

Footwear

18. Shop for shoes after you have been on your feet for a while. Feet tend to swell as the day progresses.

19. Look for shoes that you can put on and take off independently.

20. Cobblers can change shoes that buckle or tie to Velcro®-closing shoes.

21. If the tongue of the shoe keeps getting in the way, ask the cobbler to stitch it to one side of the shoe or remove it altogether.

22. Adjust the heels on your shoes by having them raised or lowered.

One time, I had a pair of dress shoes that I wanted to wear to a special event, but when I walked in them, I felt unsteady; my balance was off. I had the shoemaker take 3/8" off the heel. You couldn't even tell and it was just the adjustment I needed to comfortably and safely wear those party shoes.

23. Rub the soles of new leather shoes with sandpaper to reduce slipperiness. No sandpaper? Scrape the soles along concrete or stucco until the smooth sole surface is rough.

24. Consider replacing leather soles with rubber or crepe so that shoes are not as slippery.

25. Have the cobbler sew a leather loop at the heel that you can grab to pull on your shoe.

26. Have the eyelets enlarged to make it easier to thread the shoelaces.

27. If you're having difficulty tying your shoes, elastic shoelaces might be helpful. These laces come in a variety of styles and colors and allow you to slip your shoes on without needing to tie them. They work especially well with sneakers and athletic shoes.

28. If your feet are different sizes, or if you wear an ankle/foot orthotic (AFO) on one foot, you may need to purchase mismated shoes. Ask your local shoe store about their "split-size" or different-sized-feet policy. Many retailers, like Nordstrom, LL Bean, Birkenstock, and Healthy Feet Stores, have split-size policies; even Target gives theirs managers the option of selling split sizes on some styles. Also, try the National Odd Shoe Exchange, which deals in donated shoes (www.oddshoe.org).

29. If your feet always feel cold, wear over-the-ankle boots as slippers or look for fleece-lined or down-filled slippers.

Hosiery

30. Supersize your pantyhose.

> *Whenever I need to wear nylon hosiery, I wear queen-sized pantyhose. The leg portion is sized normally but the tummy portion is more generous than regular-sized pantyhose, which makes it easier to pull them up and down.*

31. Eliminate wearing pantyhose altogether by wearing knee-high nylon trouser socks under slacks and thigh-high stockings under dresses. Both knee-high and thigh-high stockings have elastic bands at the top to help keep them up. They are sold wherever pantyhose are sold.

32. Wearing pantyhose with a cotton crotch eliminates the need to wear underpants in addition to your hose.

33. Compression socks can be helpful when you're sedentary and sit all the time or if your feet or legs tend to swell while standing, traveling, or at the end of the day. If your feet swell, consider wearing compression socks. Compression socks range from basic support stockings to a compression level that exceeds the white antiembolism socks patients often wear in the hospital. The most aggressive compression styles require a doctor's prescription and special fitting; insurance may cover part of the cost. Order through your doctor or contact a home-health-care supply store.

For years, my feet were terribly swollen, ice cold, and painful until my physician prescribed compression socks. A fitter through a local home-health agency determined what I needed and ordered them for me. My insurance company covered the cost. Dave puts them on me before I get out of bed in the morning and takes them off when I get in bed at night. Now, my feet are normal size and are no longer cold or swollen.

34. TravelSox® uses a patented, gradual compression design to help stimulate blood flow and reduce swelling in your legs and feet. The "dress sock" look will allow you to keep your legs comfortable and energized, and your feet dry at work or play (www.arcosox.com).

35. Before you put on regular or compression socks, sprinkle powder or baking soda on your feet and between your toes.

36. Tube socks are easier to put on than socks that are shaped like a foot.

37. Look for "footies" or slipper socks with nonskid tread on the bottom to keep you steady on your feet.

38. Put a plastic bag over your foot before putting on your boots. The boots will slip on and off more easily, and your feet will stay drier longer.

Shopping

For the last 35 years, I haven't been able to shop and coordinate outfits like I used to. However, I wanted to continue to wear attractive, professional-looking clothing, so I had to find ways to adapt my old shopping techniques. By following some of the same strategies, perhaps you'll find it easier to "look good and feel better."

39. Choose clothing in colors that make you look your best.

> *One of the first things I did when my ability to shop for clothes became difficult was to have my colors analyzed by a professional color consultant. I knew some colors looked better on me than others and I wanted to spend my limited energy looking for clothes that would look good on me. Once I knew what my best colors were, I carried color swatches with me when I shopped. Then, I only looked for clothing in those colors and hues. An additional benefit was that eventually all the clothes in my closet went together and everything could be mixed and matched.*

40. Shop at clothing stores where you can receive personal attention.

> *I began shopping at small clothing stores rather than large department stores because the sales clerks seemed to have more time to help me coordinate outfits and could help me in the fitting room. The clothing cost a bit more, but the special service was worth it. I always call ahead to schedule an appointment so I have the help I need.*

41. Consider using a personal shopper. Some stores offer the services of a "personal shopper," a sales person trained to listen to your specific needs and specifications and find items you request. You can try the items on in the store with assistance from the personal shopper or take them home "on approval," where, from the convenience of your home, you can decide which products to keep and which ones to return.

42. If you are unable to go to stores to shop, shop by catalog or online. Be sure to check the return policies before you order.

*When Dave and I are invited to a special event, or I just "need"
something new "to pick me up," I use a combination of store, catalog,
Internet, and TV shopping and always find just what I want.*

43. When you arrive at an unfamiliar department store, ask where the
escalators, elevators, and restrooms are located so you can find
them easily if needed.

44. If you tend to get overheated, use the sleeves of your jacket or
sweatshirt to tie around your waist and keep your hands free.
You might also consider renting a locker—usually located near
the public restrooms.

45. Find a fitting room with a chair and sit to try on clothes. If no chair
is available, ask the sales person to get one.

46. To help determine whether a garment will fit without trying it on,
consider taking along a garment that fits you well. Ask one of the
sales staff to match the side seams and length by laying one item on
top of another.

47. Take along your measurements.

*Sometimes when I'm buying something for myself (or a family
member), I record the measurements on a piece of paper that I take with
me to the store. Then, I ask the sales person to measure the garment to
see whether it will work with the measurements. (I bring a tape measure
with me.)*

48. If trying on clothes at a store is too difficult because of your energy
level or physical disabilities, ask whether you may take the clothes
home "on approval," and try them on at your leisure.

49. If you have a friend who wears the same size as you, take this
person shopping with you and have your friend try on the
clothes. However, keep in mind that we all have different color-
ing and that colors that may look good on your friend, may not
be as flattering on you.

50. Instead of carrying your purchases around with you, have them mailed or delivered to your home.

Choosing the Right Clothing

51. Clothing made of 100% cotton will shrink and need ironing to look fresh and crisp; cotton blends with less than 50% cotton need little or no ironing. Garments made of permanent-press fabric require no ironing or special treatment. Read clothing labels before making your purchases.

52. Because they stretch, knit fabrics are easier to get on and off than woven fabrics. In addition, knit fabrics are more comfortable to sit in and do not wrinkle as much as woven fabrics.

53. Double-knit sweatpants with an elasticized waistband are particularly easy to wear and maintain.

54. When purchasing woolen coats or jackets, choose those lined with a satiny fabric. They'll be easier to put on.

55. Some fabrics are actually "heavy," meaning they have weight. Clothing made of this type of fabric may tire you out just by putting it on.

56. Where a shawl rather than a jacket with sleeves.

It's exhausting for me to put on/take off winter outerwear and I need lots of help. So, for more than 30 years, I've worn (wool and alpaca) shawls to keep warm, even during our frigid Wisconsin winters. Shawls differ in style and weight, so chose one that works for you.

57. Fabrics with a pile like velvet, corduroy, velour, and terry cloth make sliding on and off upholstered surfaces more difficult. Nylon, rayon, satin, acetates, silk, and polished cotton make sliding easier. However, your sitting stability may be compromised when you're sitting on leather or vinyl furniture.

58. If you sit a great deal, purchase garments one size larger than you normally wear. The clothing will be more comfortable to sit in and easier to put on and remove. Clothing that is too tight may actually make you feel tired. In addition, the longer length of the extra size will provide extra warmth around the ankles because the clothes will not ride up as far.

59. Consider shopping where maternity clothes are sold. The garments are generously sized and fashionable. Some of the new styles feature elastic panels hidden by pockets or a simple drawstring waistband so that no one need know they are maternity. Caftans and muumuus are loose-fitting garments that look fashionable and accommodate fluctuations in weight.

60. Short-cropped jackets, sweaters, and tops are more flattering than double-breasted garments for wheelchair users.

61. Short or three-quarter-sleeve shirts and blouses will not get caught in the spokes of a wheelchair.

62. Jackets or coats with side slits or vents are more comfortable to sit in.

63. When you find a garment you like in a style and size that fits, purchase several in colors that look good on you.

64. If you use a wheelchair full time, you may have trouble finding jeans that fit comfortably. USA Jeans are designed specifically for the seated individual. The front looks like a traditional jean, whereas the back is elastic with added fabric in the seat for comfort. Leg pockets with easy, seated access are optional. The company will customize the pants for your specific needs (www .wheelchairjeans.com).

65. Finding jeans that fit you when you don't wear a standard size is difficult.

I wear Downs Designs® Dreams/NBZ® Jeans. They're designed for people of all ages with Downs syndrome, wheelchair users, and people with differing abilities and body types. None of the jeans have buttons, snaps, or zippers; they have full elastic waistbands, belt loops, mock-fly fronts, and are made of soft and stretchy denim. The jeans are stylish and comfortable and look like the jeans everyone else is wearing. You work directly with the company, which offers a free try-on service and promises a perfect fit (877-390-4851; www.downsdesignsdreams.org).

Accessories

66. Clip-on earrings or pierced earrings on a wire that do not need a back are more practical for people who have the use of only one hand.

67. Omega-backed pierced earrings (a post with a spring clip to secure it in place) are easy to put on if you only have the use of one hand.

68. If you have trouble getting a clasp-style bracelet on or off, add an extender that lets your hand slip through the clasped bracelet. You can also use a fastening tool like the Bracelet Buddy® (www .BraceletBuddy.com).

69. Look online for videos and ideas for putting on your jewelry independently and/or making your own fasteners.

70. Customize favorite jewelry.

To make putting on necklaces and bracelets easier, I had a craft store replace the difficult-to-manage closures with magnetic clasps. Now I can put on and take off my own jewelry.

71. Necklaces that slip over your head are easier to put on and take off.

72. Keep bracelets and necklaces organized and easy to find by hanging them from hooks, a belt holder, or a store-bought necklace holder.

73. A shoulder bag worn across the body (i.e., over the head) keeps hands free and allows you to transfer the weight of your purse from your hands or shoulders to your trunk.

74. A sling-type purse/bag worn over your left shoulder puts the weight on your right hip. Slinging it over your right shoulder puts the weight on your left hip.

75. A variety of hats, neck bands, clothing, and products are available to help keep you cool. Some are filled with polymer beads that absorb water and cool you through evaporation, others use cooling tubes, misters, and cooling (fabric) technology.

76. In cold weather, wear a hooded scarf. The scarf portion will keep the neck warm, and when not in use, the hood hangs securely around your neck, leaving your hands free for other things.

77. Rather than wearing a scarf with ends that you have to wrap around your neck several times, purchase a mobius (endless loop) style that will slip over your head.

78. Wear mittens rather than gloves.

When I could no longer put on gloves, I purchased mittens with a wide, unrestricted opening so I could simply slip my hand inside.

79. For folks whose hands are contracted into a fist, an oven mitt may be easier to put on to provide protection from the cold.

Simple Clothing Alterations

80. When you put on a jacket or sweater, keep long-sleeved shirts from bunching up at the elbows by sewing loops inside the cuffs. Just grab onto a loop as you put your arm into the second garment and tuck the loop up into the shirtsleeve when you're done. You could also sew loops of bias tape inside the waistband of slacks and trousers. Use the loops to pull pants up and down.

81. Attach a small pendant, locket, key chain object, or notebook ring to the zipper-pull on a jacket or sweater to make it easier to grasp.

82. Enlarge buttonholes and replace small buttons with larger buttons. Textured buttons are easier to manage than smooth ones.

83. Use Velcro to replace buttons and other fasteners. Sew an existing buttonhole closed and sew the button on top of it. Then sew the soft fuzzy side of the Velcro on the underside of the closed-up buttonhole. Sew the other piece of Velcro, the hard side with the small hooks, where the button used to be.

84. Sew buttons on with elastic thread. If buttoned cuff openings are too small to get your fist through, move the buttons to make the opening larger. Or, you can sew the buttons on with elastic thread, which will give the re-buttoned cuff opening an extra quarter inch or so of wiggle room.

85. Purchase a buttonhook or make one by using a large safety pin. To button, hook one of the buttons with the closed safety pin. Then thread the safety pin through the buttonhole, and the button will follow. You may also try opening up a metal paper clip and using one of the hooked ends to "catch" the button.

86. Use Velcro or zippers to create openings in the side seams or inseams in your slacks or trousers. They will be easier to put on and take off. To make skirts easier to put on and take off, open the back seam and sew in Velcro to keep the skirt seams together. The same technique may be possible on some dresses. Velcro may be unsatisfactory in seams that take a lot of stress; in these situations, replace short zippers with longer zippers to make openings larger.

87. If you are unable to make these simple alterations to your clothing, consider hiring someone to make the alterations or ask your laundry or dry cleaners if they can recommend someone.

Clothing Resources

Adaptive-Clothing Retailers

Clothing for people who are seated is much different than that designed for individuals who walk. For more options, search online for "adaptive clothing or apparel," "clothing for people with disabilities," or "clothing for people in wheelchairs."

www.AdaptationsbyAdrian.com
www.BuckandBuck.com
www.downsdesignsdreams.org
www.EasyAccessClothing.com
www.IZCollection.com
www.Janska.com
www.silverts.com
www.wheelchairjeans.com

It's a delicate balancing act to manage living with MS. To help you find a variety of adaptive-clothing retailers, look in the Resource section of this book. It is my hope that these tips and strategies will help you look your very best.

CHAPTER 12

Working

In our society, having a job and working is part of the American culture, so when the effects of multiple sclerosis begin to affect your ability to work, it can be very stressful and emotional. I know how difficult it was for me.

Ever since I was in high school and befriended some girls who were deaf, I wanted to be a teacher of the deaf. I was passionate about my work; it was part of who I was. So, when my mobility and my ability to sign and fingerspell were affected, it was devastating for me and for my career.

This was in 1979, before any of the disease-modifying therapies had been discovered. Thankfully, with today's treatments for MS, many people continue to work with only minor adjustments. Others, like me, may go from diagnosis to having to give up their job relatively quickly.

At first, I didn't tell anyone at work about my MS; I "tried to pass" as normal. But it was difficult to keep up my normal pace. Thankfully, by this time in my career, I was working with the teachers and other educational professionals and had more control over my daily schedule. I began to make simple workplace modifications that didn't involve my employer.

Simple Workplace Modifications

1. Arrange your space so that everything you need is within arm's reach.

2. Conserve your energy by keeping heavy books or binders that you use frequently near you rather than on a shelf or in a bookcase.

3. Put the most frequently used files in the lower drawers of your desk or filing cabinet, so you can reach them from a seated position.

4. Consider wearing wrist braces (off-the-shelf at pharmacies) or "massaging" ergonomic gloves, if you do a lot of keyboarding.

5. Bring a pillow to sit on or to use as lumbar support.

6. Use a footstool to rest your feet on.

7. Bring a fan to keep you cool.

8. Purchase a rubber floor mat to stand on if you stand a lot.

9. A desk lamp might provide better and more direct lighting than overhead lighting fixtures.

10. If the noise from other cubicles makes it difficult to concentrate, a fan or computer playing soft music might help. At times, headphones or foam earplugs may be necessary.

11. Take frequent short breaks to rest your mind and body. If you need a reminder to take a break, there are many apps that can help you set up a schedule that works for you.

12. Get up and move. Go for a walk, get a drink, or use the bathroom. Go talk to coworkers at their desks rather than using the phone or e-mail.

13. Change your position frequently. Stretch your arms above your head, move your neck—tip it forward and to both sides to loosen tight muscles—or stand up and move your legs.

14. Write yourself a reminder.

    Before I left the office for the weekend or on vacation, I'd write myself a "where to start" message. That way, when I returned to the office I knew exactly where I left off and could get back to work faster.

Disclosing Your Disability

If the accommodations you've made are not adequate for your increasing needs, you may want to consider disclosing your diagnosis to your boss. The decision to disclose (or not disclose) your MS is deeply personal and one that needs careful consideration. (Even the most supportive employers can become less supportive when they think your work product will be affected.)

When my limitations became more visible and I couldn't hide them anymore, I decided to tell my boss. I was clear and unemotional as I told him about my MS diagnosis and how it affected me. He listened and was more supportive than I thought he would be. Then I told everyone else; I wanted people to hear about the diagnosis from me. I wanted to avoid gossip and misinformation.

Here are some things to consider before disclosing your condition:

15. Talk about your job-related issues and concerns with a knowledgeable person who can help you process your decision. The Job Accommodation Network (JAN) provides free, confidential consulting services for people with physical or intellectual limitations that affect employment. They offer one-on-one consultation about job accommodation ideas, request and negotiate accommodations, and your rights under the Americans with Disabilities Act (ADA). Find them online at www.askjan.org or call 800-526-7234 (voice) or 877-781-9403 (TTY).

16. Every state in the United States is required to provide vocational rehabilitation (VR) services for people who have disabilities and work. These services include helping you and your employer fund workplace accommodations, find or maintain transportation for getting to work, and overcome other challenges you may face to continue working with a chronic illness like MS. How each state administers its programs may be different, so search online for "vocational rehabilitation services" (and your state) to find out what services are offered and how to access them.

17. The ADA states that employees with disabilities and chronic conditions are entitled to a reasonable accommodation, that is, a reasonable adjustment to a job or work environment that makes it possible for an individual with a disability to perform job duties. If your employer employs 15 people or more, the employer is required to make "reasonable accommodations" by the ADA. To learn more, visit www.ada.gov/employment.

Determining What You Need

Because it's the employee's responsibility to ask for the accommodations he or she needs, it's important that you determine what modifications or accommodations would be most helpful to you (and have an idea of what they might cost).

18. Ask your doctor for a referral to a physiatrist (a doctor who specializes in physical medicine and rehabilitation) and/or a physical/occupational therapist. These medical professionals can do a full assessment of your limitations and abilities, provide tips for working smarter, and advise and give you valuable information and/or recommendations on products (chairs, desks, computer setup, glasses, repetitive-strain programs, etc.) that could be helpful.

19. AbleData provides objective information about assistive technology devices (www.abledata.com). Search "workplace."

20. Microsoft Accessibility Resource Centers, located in many U.S. states (and around the world), have knowledgeable staff that can show you how to use computer accessibility features and how to select assistive technology products that are right for you (www.microsoft.com/enable).

21. The National Council on Independent Living provides a directory to your local Independent Living Center, where you will find assessment, assistance, and resources to solutions to overcome your limitations (www.ncil.org).

22. Two US government websites, www.Disability.gov and www .dol.gov/odep, provide information regarding issues about working when you have a disability. There are also links to states and financial loan programs.

23. A reasonable accommodation will differ for each person. Think about what might make working easier for you.

24. The effects of your illness or medications you take might make it necessary for you to come in to work earlier or later or to reduce your hours and work part time instead of full time.

25. If your job requires a lot of standing or your job is too physical for you to continue doing, ask for a reassignment of duties to a less demanding position.

26. Discuss being retrained to do another job in the workplace that is less physically or mentally demanding. VR services may pay for the training or classes you need.

27. If the day comes when you are "no longer able to do your job," even with reasonable accommodation, you may need to look for a different career. If you need job-placement services, to learn different skills, or have additional training, your state VR agency can help defray the cost.

Your attitude is important. When asking your employer for any kind of job accommodation, remember that working with him or her to find a mutually beneficial solution is better for everyone than demanding your rights under the law.

Working From Home

If you have established a good reputation for diligence and a good work ethic with your employer, you may request to work part or all of the time at home in order to save energy or meet your need for frequent rest periods or energy fluctuations.

28. Many technological advances, like videoconferencing and document scanners, along with e-mail and texting, can even connect a global workforce. You will need to work with your employer to establish your work hours and to create a way to evaluate your work product.

29. Working from home is an adjustment, especially if you've been used to going out to work.

When I retired from teaching at the age of 35, I had to make lots of changes and now I love the convenience. My office commute is 20 seconds. I don't have to venture out in minus 20° weather, and I can crank up the heat or air conditioning, so I'm always comfortable. The kitchen serves all my favorite foods and the bathroom is always available and accessible. And, if a deadline has me panicked, there's always ice cream in the freezer to calm my nerves.

Creating a Dedicated Workspace

30. Plan your workspace to accommodate your needs now and in the future. Your state's VR services can be helpful in the process.

31. Desk surfaces should be 24 to 28 inches in depth, any deeper and a seated person cannot reach them.

32. When possible, allow a 5-foot turning radius for a mobility device.

33. Make doorways as wide as possible, 36 inches is the best.

34. Consider using folding or sliding doors on closets.

35. Storage areas, shelves, and file cabinets are easier to manage if they are at least 12 inches off the floor and no higher than 54 inches. Lateral file cabinets are easiest to use by most people.

36. Plug your computer, monitor, printer, and so on, into an easy-to-reach, multiple-outlet power strip and turn all the devices on or off by pressing one switch. You can find power strips with safety features, such as circuit breakers or surge protectors, at hardware and discount stores.

Computer Technology

37. Computers offer many built-in accessibility features to make using the computer possible for people with limited physical or sensory abilities. On your computer, you can check out the accessibility options in the control panel.

38. Different types of keyboard configurations allow you to type if you have a limited range of motion.

39. Screen enlargers enhance the picture from your computer monitor if your vision is limited.

40. Screen-reading software reads aloud whatever text is displayed on the screen (for example, the newspaper downloaded from the Internet).

41. Voice-activated, speech-recognition programs, such as Dragon® Naturally Speaking, enable you to speak your thoughts directly onto the computer screen, dramatically reducing the time spent typing on a keyboard.

Telephones

42. To make holding a standard phone receiver easier, use a shoulder rest.

43. Use a speakerphone.

44. Purchase an inexpensive headset at an office-supply store to keep your hands free. It's a headband with a microphone and earphone attached.

45. Be sure to try out the buttons on phones before you buy. Some are easier to press than others. In addition, consider the weight and shape of the receiver; they vary greatly from model to model.

46. Look for amplified telephones with a "talk-back" feature that repeats the digits aloud after each key-press.

47. Preprogram your telephone to eliminate the need to dial frequently used numbers.

48. If you have difficulty hearing or understanding conversation on the telephone, a captioned telephone shows the caller's message on a screen as one speaks, much like closed-captioning on televisions. You need a landline or a high-speed Internet connection to use this device. For more information, visit www.CapTel.com or www.CaptionCallPhone.com.

49. Cordless telephones allow you to move the telephone to all parts of the room or house; however, they do not work when the electricity goes out, so make sure that you have a hardwired phone or cell phone for emergencies.

50. If you have trouble locating telephones with the features you need, contact your local phone company's special-needs center.

51. Set your cellular phone to silent and let calls go to voice mail or let an answering machine pick up calls, so you can screen phone calls or take messages while you rest.

52. Cellular phones have many accessibility features, such as hands-free and voice commands, built in. Ask your carrier to explain, demonstrate, and program your phone for the features most useful to you.

53. If you need additional features to make using your smartphone easier, there is probably an app for that. Ask your carrier representative to show you how to search your phone's app-store feature for what you are looking for. Search online for similar apps available for tablets and computers.

54. Remember: If you need a work-related piece of equipment, software, an accessibility modification, and telephones, contact your state Department of Vocational Rehabilitation to help defray the costs.

Other Thoughts on Working From Home

55. Dress the part.

> *I get up, get dressed, and put on my makeup and earrings as if I were going out to work. I never wear jeans or a sweatshirt because I can't get into a work mind-set when I wear "play" clothes. Also, if someone drops by or I have an appointment with my accountant, computer consultant, or printer, I want to look like the professional I am.*

56. Have a routine. Set work hours and keep to a schedule, whenever possible.

57. Work when your energy is best and you can focus, even if it's late at night.

58. During your "rest time," put your feet up, meditate, or take a nap.

59. If your friends and neighbors call during work hours, cut social conversations short by asking the caller when you can return the call.

60. Keep the TV off. It's too easy to fritter away an hour or 2. If there's something on during the day that you don't want to miss, record the program to watch later.

61. Seek opportunities to be with people. Working from home can be very solitary and isolating. Schedule lunch meetings, take a class, attend a conference, or join a professional group as a way of stimulating your creative juices and improving your skills.

When You Can No Longer Work

62. If you have a work history; have paid into Social Security; and have physical, sensory, cognitive, or mental limitations as a result of MS that make it impossible for you to work, apply for Social

Security Disability Insurance (SSDI). Your dependent children may qualify to receive benefits as well. Review the qualifications and benefits at www.SSA.gov/disability. You can also get a free disability qualification evaluation at www.disability-benefits-help.org.

63. Your doctor, who knows and understands your condition as well as your limitations, can be an advocate and provide evidence to support your case.

64. Keep a log of all your interactions with the Social Security Administration, VR counselors, doctors, and occupational/physical therapists, including the full name, date of contact, phone numbers, and what was said. Start a file and keep copies of everything (documents, reports, test results, evaluations, etc.).

65. Entities, such as the National MS Society and veteran's groups, have local support groups and counselors to provide guidance; they may even help you fill out the forms.

66. Be honest about ALL your limitations (cognitive, sensory, and physical), as well as your symptoms. Don't leave anything out or "sugar-coat" your problems. It is not about what you CAN do on a good day; it is all about what you CAN'T do on a bad day. Remember, all the reviewer has to go on is what is on the forms; he or she cannot see your pain or your inability to think or move. Tell it like it is.

67. Don't be surprised if you're turned down the first time you apply for benefits; most people are. You know you can't work, so appeal the decision, even if it takes several years and multiple appeals.

68. Disability appeals are denied at an even higher rate than initial applications. So, if you are denied, hire an attorney who specializes in Social Security Disability law. Every state has lawyers who represent people who have been denied disability benefits; consult your state Bar Association for a list of attorneys with this specialty.

69. Hiring an attorney will not cost you anything. When you win your appeal and receive benefits, the lawyer receives a onetime payment (a percentage set by law) of your disability benefit and you receive the rest. If you lose, there still is no cost to you. Using legal counsel can increase your chances of receiving benefits significantly.

70. Don't give up!!! Even if you feel unwell and discouraged because you cannot work, hang in there and fight for yourself and for your benefits. You have paid into the Social Security system when you worked specifically for this reason. Receiving benefits because of your disability is your right.

I encourage you to adapt, modify, reorganize, and recreate a workplace environment that makes your job easier. Use the resources, services, and products in this chapter to help you continue to work.

CHAPTER 13

Driving and Disability

As my multiple sclerosis progressed, my ability to drive safely became a serious concern. My reaction time had slowed and it affected my ability to move my foot quickly from the gas to the brake. I did not want to risk having an accident, so I voluntarily gave up driving. I was only 39.

I share my personal thoughts on giving up driving and how I handled finding rides in Chapters 2 to 14.

If you feel your ability to drive is being affected, you may find these tips helpful.

Evaluating Your Abilities

1. Contact your doctor, occupational therapist, or a trained driver rehabilitation specialist about getting a professional driving evaluation to determine whether it is still safe for you to drive.

2. A driving evaluation consists of both a clinical and a behind-the-wheel assessment, which will include your physical function, visual acuity, your ability to process information quickly, and your reaction time. In addition, you'll learn what kinds of vehicle modifications or adaptations (such as hand controls) might make it easier and safer for you to drive.

3. To find an evaluator and motor vehicle adaptation choices for people with disabilities, visit the National Highway Transportation and Safety Administration website (www.nhtsa.gov) and review

their free brochure, "Adapting Motor Vehicles for People With Disabilities."

4. To find a driver rehabilitation specialist in your community, the Association for Driver Rehabilitation Specialists (www.aded.net) provides a list of dealers by state.

5. If your employment requires that you need a vehicle to get to, from, or for work, contact your state vocational rehabilitation agency. This agency is charged with helping people with disabilities obtain and retain employment. A counselor from the agency will evaluate your ability to work, help you draw up a plan to keep working, arrange for necessary evaluations, and possibly fund all or part of the adaptations necessary for your vehicle. See Chapter 12 for more workplace accommodations.

6. Every state has its own rules regarding who qualifies for disabled license plates or placards, and what benefits having them gives you. Most usually provide designated, free-parking spots for people with disabilities; often someone with disabled plates/placards can exceed the time limit on meters and get full-service fuel for the self-service price at certain gas stations. Consult your state's Department of Motor Vehicles or follow the quick links at www.DMV.org.

Making Your Vehicle More Accessible

In the last few years, many vehicle modifications and adapted equipment choices have become available. Some are standard features or add-ons installed by the car manufacturer or an automotive mobility dealer. Others are low-cost, easy-to-install products that are readily available online, at a pharmacy, or at a home-health or discount store near you.

Getting In and Out of Your Vehicle

7. A portable trapeze-style handle strap goes around the top of your vehicle's window frame and provides a cushion grip to help you pull yourself up and out of the car. The device is fully adjustable

for maximum support, regardless of your height. It works on any vehicle with a door frame; the strap is not suitable for convertibles or other vehicles without an enclosed window. Versions of this device may be marketed as Car Caddie or Able Life Auto Assist Handle.

8. A car door-latch grab bar is a superstrong personal support handle that helps you get in or out of the car with ease. The removable bar inserts into your door's latch to give extra leverage for maneuvering, lowering yourself into the car, or standing up. Some are constructed of steel, others of aluminum. Most have a soft nonslip grip handle. They can be used on either the driver or passenger side and are compact enough to store in your glove box. Some models will safely support up to 500 pounds and may be used in an emergency to break a window or cut a seat belt. Available under names such as Handybar®, Car Cane™, and Beyoung® Car Door Assist.

You may wish to use the devices listed in 7 and 8 together.

9. If you have trouble sliding into a car with upholstered seats, try tucking a vinyl tablecloth or a plastic garbage bag into the seat. That way, you'll create a surface that's slippery enough to slide on.

10. A commercially made "slick sliding pad" provides nearly effortless sliding and rotation on and off of a car seat. The 18" × 22" mat provides a bit of cushion on the seat, stays flat and is comfortable to sit upon; designed with six sections, it folds up easily to carry with you for use on any seat, anywhere.

11. Transfer swivel seats or disks allow you to turn yourself, or a passenger with a disability, to allow getting into and out of the car without twisting.

Simple Adaptations to Your Car

12. A seat belt extender is a piece of seat belt material about 8 inches long, with a buckle on the end that clicks into the existing seat belt.

Originally designed to provide extra room for larger drivers and passengers over 215 pounds, it makes the seat belt easier to grasp, pull, and buckle for people with arm, shoulder, or strength limitations. Unfortunately, seat belt extenders are not a universal fit, so check with your dealer to see whether they are available for your vehicle.

13. If you find wearing a seat belt is uncomfortable because of sensitive skin, body pain, or a pacemaker, a leather, vinyl, or sheepskin seat belt cover will cushion the pressure of the belt against your neck and chest and make driving or riding more comfortable.

14. If you have trouble turning your head to see cars in your blind spot, install panoramic or wide-angle rear and side-view mirrors to widen your view. You will find that when using the regular and wide-angle mirrors together, you'll have greater visibility and won't have to turn your neck as much. Some mirrors have double-sided tape on the back of them, so they're easy to install; others attach with screws. Look for these mirrors where automotive accessories are sold.

15. Adaptive key devices are enlarged ergonomic handles that fit on your regular key and give better leverage to make turning keys easier. Hardware stores and home health care stores have different styles from which to choose. Be sure to try before you buy to see which works best for you.

16. Remote car starters not only make it possible to start your car without having to twist a key, but, if you are especially sensitive to hot or cold temperatures, you can start your vehicle, turn on the heater or air conditioner, defrost the windows, and even turn on the car lights from your home or office. You may choose to install the starter yourself or have it professionally installed. Search for these devices online or at automotive, discount, or big-box stores.

17. If you need to restrict car use by someone with cognitive MS problems, consider installing an automotive battery-disconnect switch to

the car battery. With just the turn of a knob, you can quickly disconnect and reconnect power to the battery. The device is easy to install and works on cars, trucks, boats, and recreational vehicles (RVs). It's designed to affect starting only and will not affect the clock, the radio, or computer settings.

Professionally Installed Vehicle Modifications

18. Your driver rehabilitation specialist can recommend a mobility equipment dealer to make modifications to your vehicle. Or you can contact the National Mobility Equipment Dealers Association (NMEDA) directly; they will be able to connect you with dealers in your community (www.NMEDA.com).

19. Dealers will be able to educate you on the type of vehicle adaptions that are possible and show you wheelchair-accessible vehicles that will meet your specific transportation needs. Some dealers offer their own programs to help fund vehicle modifications, whereas others will help you locate possible funding sources.

Moderately Priced Modifications

There are a wide variety of products to make it easier and safer for you to drive your current vehicle. Here are just a few:

20. Add a turning knob to the steering wheel to make it easier to grip and turn the wheel with the use of just one hand.

21. Raise the foot pedals to make it easier for you to reach.

22. Install a left-foot accelerator pedal if your right foot/leg is weak.

23. Install hand controls if you find you cannot operate the foot pedals.

24. Install turn signal extenders.

More Costly Options

If you are considering purchasing a vehicle, there are many types of vehicles (cars, trucks, minivans, utility vehicles, vans, RVs, even vehicles used on a farm) that can be made accessible, whether you are a driver or only a passenger. Consider the following:

25. Wheelchair or scooter lifts

26. Wheelchair security systems (e.g., special brake locks on the wheels of your wheelchair)

27. Electric transfer seat bases that allow an individual to move from his or her wheelchair or scooter to the driver's seat

28. Wheelchair or scooter carriers, allowing the chair or scooter to be transported

29. Alternative steering in the form of hand controls

30. Vehicles that allow side or rear entry

31. Raised car or van door tops

32. Dropped vehicle floors

33. Power-based ramps that allow for wheelchair or scooter entry

Transportation Services

Public transportation, service organizations, faith communities, and friends can help you create your own network of people who can help you safely get you where you need to go.

34. If you live in a city with bus service, most buses are equipped with kneeling technology that lowers the bus down so a person using a mobility device (cane, crutches, walker, or wheelchair) can get on and off more easily. Usually the first few rows of seats are reserved for people with disabilities and some buses even have seats that fold out of the way so a wheelchair can fit instead. A companion may accompany you at no cost.

35. The Americans with Disabilities Act (ADA) requires that door-to-door transportation (paratransit) be provided for people who cannot use regular fixed-route bus services. Unlike regular buses that run on a regular schedule; paratransit usually needs to be reserved a day or two in advance. Contact your local bus company for more information and to see whether you qualify for this service. Your doctor's documentation of your sensitivity to hot, cold, or other weather conditions may prove to be all the proof you need.

36. Accessible taxi services provide taxis equipped with ramps for people with disabilities. Because accessible taxis comprise only a small percentage of the fleet, you might have a longer wait for a ride than with a traditional taxi.

37. Medicaid recipients can take nonemergency taxi transportation to health care appointments, including medical tests and doctor's appointments, for a small fee. Contact your case manager or county social services agency for more information.

38. Assisted Transportation Systems provide rides along with hands-on assistance (opening doors, physical support, verbal guidance, etc.) to people with disabilities. These are often private service agencies, some are subsidized and low cost, and others are not. Fees may vary, so inquire before you ride.

39. Disabled American Veterans, support groups, and service organizations that cater to the elderly often have volunteers who provide rides for people who do not drive but are ambulatory enough to get in and out of a vehicle, whether or not they use a wheelchair or walker. There is usually a fee.

40. Cheaper than a taxi, if you are able to get in and out of a regular vehicle, rides services like Uber and Lift may be helpful in getting you from here to there quickly. Make sure you inquire about the driver's vehicle in advance, so you know you can get in and out easily.

41. For a list of accessible transportation services in your area, contact your county social services agency, Aging and Disability Resource Center (ADRC), or call the United Way hotline at 2-1-1.

CHAPTER 14

Weekend Getaways and Extended Travel

Sometimes a change of scenery and getting away is the pick-me-up I need. However, when you live with multiple sclerosis (MS), it's so much easier to "stay put." Changing daily routines and leaving the comforts of home requires energy we don't have and can present unexpected challenges. However, I found that with some preplanning and a spirit of adventure, I can relax and enjoy a weekend getaway or a major family vacation, just like everyone else. I share tips and examples here in hopes that they'll take some of the anxiety and guesswork out of traveling and give you the confidence and encouragement you need to get out and get away.

Planning Your Trip

1. Do research online and/or contact agencies (Department of Tourism, Convention and Visitors' Bureau, Chamber of Commerce) to collect information about the places you wish to visit; these offices can send you brochures and provide information on accessibility, attractions, accommodations, restaurants, and so on.

2. If you choose to work with a travel agent, find one who has experience working with travelers with special needs. There usually is no charge for their services. In fact, you'll often save money, because travel agents know about special rates and tour packages. Whether you make the reservations yourself or work with a travel agent, always be completely honest about your needs.

3. Some travel agencies focus on travelers with medical issues and/or disabilities. Some agencies even help arrange for companions to accompany you and provide special-needs support while you travel.

4. The International Association for Medical Assistance to Travelers (IAMAT) is a nonprofit organization that provides important information to travelers with medical concerns. Travelers can obtain a directory of English-speaking doctors in foreign countries. Updated each year, the directory lists doctors who have had training in the United States, Great Britain, or Canada. IAMAT also has world immunization charts, malaria risk charts, and world climate charts, and can tell you about the food and water in the countries you plan to visit.

5. The Society for Accessible Travel and Hospitality (SATH) is a nonprofit organization that acts as a clearinghouse for accessible tourism information worldwide. They are in contact with organizations in many countries to promote the development of facilities for people with disabilities (http://sath.org).

Choosing a Hotel or Motel

6. Accessibility standards may vary from state to state, but, in general, newly constructed or recently remodeled buildings have the best facilities for travelers with disabilities. Older motels or hotels may not be accessible. Accessible rooms are generally larger than regular rooms and have large bathrooms with a raised toilet and grab bars by the toilet and inside the tub and/or shower. Light switches usually are lower and doorway openings are wider. In addition to regular smoke alarms, accessible rooms often have flashing lights to alert hearing-impaired guests in case of fire.

7. Ask specific questions when making your reservations. How wide are the doorways? Does the handicapped room have a tub or roll-in shower? Is there a fold-down seat in the shower stall? If no shower seat is provided, do they have a shower chair you may use during your stay? How high are the beds? (Some hotel beds are so high off the floor that they are impossible for some people to manage.)

8. If climbing stairs is a problem, request a room on a lower floor, near stairways and exits. Remember that elevators may not be used in a fire emergency.

9. If you make hotel reservations through a toll-free number, be aware that the operator will not be able to answer your specific accessibility questions. You will have to call the hotel directly. If you require a "handicapped" room, ask how you can ensure that the room will be held until you arrive.

10. Most hotels are willing to make accommodations for guests. Can they provide an extension cord to plug in your wheelchair, distilled water for your continuous positive airway pressure (CPAP) machine, or remove furniture if the room is too crowded for mobility?

11. If you have asthma, allergies, or chemical sensitivities, clean air in your hotel room is a must. When you make your hotel reservations, ask whether they have hypoallergenic rooms or if they can treat your room with an ozone machine to knock out scents and pollen before you arrive. If the answer to both is "no," you may need to select a different hotel, one that can accommodate your needs.

12. If you require a mini fridge to keep your medications cool, be advised that if you have a mini fridge delivered to your room, they often turn the thermostat up to high and it can freeze whatever you put inside. Be sure to check the temperature before you store items in a hotel mini frig.

13. Select a hotel that is centrally located to the areas you plan to visit; you don't want to waste time and energy traveling from one side of town to another.

14. If the hotel you choose has a concierge, consider contacting him or her prior to your visit and ask that he or she put together a packet of tourist information for the dates of your visit. The concierge will also be able to make restaurant reservations, obtain theater tickets, and get tickets for the sights that you want to see. (Sometimes they have "connections" and can make arrangements for you that you couldn't make for yourself.)

15. In "all-suites" hotels, guest rooms are two-room suites. As you enter, there's a sitting room with a couch that converts into a queen-sized bed, a table, and a kitchenette. There's a separate bedroom and the bathroom is off the hallway that separates the two rooms. While someone naps in the bedroom, others may watch TV, play cards, or have a snack. In addition, those who need to refrigerate medication or carefully monitor their diet will find the microwave, refrigerator, and sink more of a necessity than a convenience. Guests are invited to bring in their own food and beverages. Many "all-suites" hotels serve a complimentary breakfast each morning.

16. In a "residence" hotel, there's a fully equipped kitchen, including a stove, refrigerator, dishwasher, garbage disposal, pots, pans, dishes, and so on. Some hotel chains have a grocery-shopping service for guests and will fill the cabinets and refrigerator with requested items. Some "residence inns" may serve a complimentary breakfast as well.

Getting Ready for Your Trip

I'm a list maker; it's the only way I can keep all the details of my life under my control. I use my travel-related lists time after time to keep me organized and reduce my stress when preparing for a trip. When seasons, destinations, and our family's needs change, I amend and revise the lists.

Your Packing List

To avoid forgetting "something," I created a master packing list so I can check off items as I pack them. When I finish packing, I put the list in the suitcase so that when I repack for the trip home, I don't leave anything behind. (Laminating the list makes it more durable.)

The list contains all the obvious major categories: clothing, accessories, toiletries, medications, insurance cards, trip-specific information (photo ID/passport, itinerary, tickets, and handicapped parking placard), devices (chargers, cords, memory cards, earphones, camera, etc.), and "fun stuff" (games, playing cards, reading material, sporting equipment, etc.).

17. Whenever you travel, take a copy of your driver's license, passport, insurance cards, and medication prescriptions. To be even safer, take two copies of each and have a companion carry one copy, while you carry a copy of his or her information.

18. If you travel with your spouse or a companion, consider packing a change of clothes in each other's bag, just in case your luggage is lost or delayed.

The following are additional items you may want on your list. Including them on your list will also remind you of any items you need to purchase before you leave.

19. Purchase trial-size bottles and tubes of everything from deodorant and hair spray to toothpaste and hand creams; you may prefer to purchase empty travel-size bottles that you can fill with your own toiletries.

20. Hand sanitizer and wet wipes are not just for your hands. You'll use them to wipe down airplane tray tables, your wheelchair steering mechanism and armrests, and other items that come in contact with dirty hands and unclean environments.

21. Pack a second pair of eyeglasses. Take the prescription for your eyeglasses, as well. If they are lost or damaged, you usually can have a replacement pair made in a short time.

22. Bring paper maps, especially if you have trouble reading digital screens. You may even want to enlarge the route to your destination or to points of interest on a photocopy machine.

23. Consider a magnifying glass if you have difficulty reading standard print. Handheld magnifiers fit in your pocket or purse and will enlarge print on menus, brochures, and tourist information.

24. A bent-neck straw will make drinking a glass of water easier while lying in bed.

25. You may need a reacher to help you retrieve items you drop on the floor or have been pushed into the middle of a table or the back of the closet. There are dozens of reachers on the market. Some have a locking grip, a hook, a sticky pad, or a small magnet on the end. Some "telescope" to allow you to change the length. Some have a light at the tip and some fold in half. Check online to find the types of reachers currently available and to read the product details.

26. If you are traveling with powered devices, such as a cell phone, computer, air cleaner, CPAP machine, or power wheelchair, you may want to take an extension cord with you to make sure that you are able to use outlets that may be out of your reach. Oftentimes, the convenient power outlets are already taken with lamps, phones, radio alarm clocks, and other devices.

27. If you have a number of items to plug in each night, pack a power strip.

28. If you have difficulty with fine motor movements, consider taking along a pair of needle-nose pliers to use to adjust the thermostat, turn on a lamp, or unzip your suitcase.

29. A few spring-type clothespins will close the gap in hotel room drapes to keep the light out.

30. Hotel bed pillows vary widely in size, shape, and weight. If you are concerned about having trouble sleeping because the pillow "isn't right," consider taking your special pillow with you.

I ALWAYS travel with my small, crib-sized pillow.

31. Bring a small, freestanding mirror to help you put on your makeup and fix your hair. Sometimes hotel mirrors are difficult to get close to, especially for people who use wheelchairs.

Because my hands are too weak to wring out a washcloth, I always travel with a thin washcloth that I know I can use. I take a small plastic bag with me for those instances when I have to pack up before the cloth is dry.

32. When you fly, consider packing a small neck pillow in your carry-on luggage. An inflatable pillow is easier to pack and transport than a microbead or foam pillow.

33. Consider packing a brief statement from your physician regarding your medical history, including the nature of your disability/disabilities, allergies to medications, and current treatment plans, including your prescriptions and other important health details.

34. If you are traveling overseas, take a photocopy of your passport and two passport photos with you and keep them separate from your passport. Then, if your passport is lost or stolen, you will have what you need to replace it.

35. Whenever and wherever you travel, you always have to be prepared for unexpected emergencies and delays, like severe weather conditions, natural disasters, or other unforeseen circumstances. That means taking an adequate supply of prescription medications and over-the-counter remedies with you. You may want to carry a doctor's prescription in your wallet or have your prescriptions filled at a pharmacy that uses a computer network. Also, take along your doctor's phone number. That way, if there's a problem filling the prescription, or you have a medical emergency or problem on the trip, you will be able to contact your doctor easily.

36. If you travel by air with a power wheelchair, scooter, or other important piece of equipment, tag all parts with your name, address, and telephone number, so that they will not get lost if the equipment must be disassembled to fit into the cargo hold. As an added safety precaution, take along a copy of the assembly instructions in case you need them when you arrive at your destination.

A Few Days Before You Leave

37. Create a list of items that you need to take care of before you go on a trip.

My list has changed over the years and has included getting substitute drivers for carpools; canceling lessons; making arrangements for pets; canceling salt delivery, pest control, food deliveries, and so on. Other items on the list could include finding someone to water the plants, mow the lawn/shovel the snow, canceling newspaper/mail delivery, or arranging for someone to take in the mail for you. Refill your prescriptions and purchase over-the-counter medications (aspirin, cortisone cream, antibiotic ointments, laxatives, cold tablets, cough drops, etc.), vitamins, and sunscreen. Return books to the library. Get small bills and change for tips and tolls. Leave a house key and itinerary (with phone numbers) with your neighbor. Contact your credit card company to let them know that you will be traveling so that your purchases will not raise suspicion that your card was stolen.

38. For car trips: Check the air in the tires, including the spare. Purchase snack foods for the cooler. Put selected tools and an emergency kit in the trunk for unexpected situations.

39. Rent a wheelchair or scooter. If your travel destination will involve lots of walking, consider taking a wheelchair with you. You can rent wheelchairs from some pharmacies, home health supply, or rental stores. Or consider renting the mobility device at your destination. Some local businesses may deliver the mobility device directly to your hotel and pick it up after you leave.

40. A few days before you leave, call the hotel to confirm your reservation. And, if you are going to arrive late, tell the staff to make a note of it on your reservation so they don't give your room away.

One time Dave and I arrived at a (newly built) hotel to find that the "handicapped room" we had reserved was NOT accessible. I couldn't even get into the bathroom because the doorway was too narrow. We called down to the front desk and asked how this could be. Then we were told that they HAD put us in a "handicapped room," a "hearing" handicapped room. All their wheelchair-accessible rooms were filled so they thought it wouldn't matter. Fortunately, they rectified the situation by putting us in a (large, handicapped) suite, at no extra charge.

41. Confirm your airline reservations.

42. Make certain that your airline ticket, frequent flier account, and passport have the same exact spelling of your name.

Before You Walk Out the Door

43. Have a list of tasks to do immediately before you leave. Set timer lights. Turn down the thermostat and hot water heater. (We always turn off the water to our house.) Grind up anything left in the garbage disposal and take out the garbage. Flush toilets. Check to see that electric blankets, curling iron, stove, oven, and coffee maker are turned off. Check to see that all the doors and windows are locked. Set the house alarm if you have one.

Luggage and Travel Accessories

44. Luggage, briefcase, musical instrument, and so on, are easier to carry if you add a soft, cushioned handle and/or shoulder strap made of neoprene gel. Put brightly colored ribbon, luggage tags, or duct tape on your luggage to make it stand out so it is easy to identify.

45. Be sure to put your home or business address and phone number on each piece of luggage, including your carry-ons. Put the same information inside your luggage as well. If your luggage is lost or stolen and recovered later, the airline will deliver it to your home free of charge.

46. If you carry a purse, computer bag, or special pillows when you travel, consider taking these items in bright colors. You'll have a better chance of seeing them as you exit a cab, courtesy van, plane, or restaurant. (Dark colors tend to blend in and "disappear" in the fast pace of moving from one place to another.)

47. It's easier to navigate the narrow airplane aisles when you aren't pulling a carry-on bag. Consider using a backpack as your carry-on bag. The weight of the bag is distributed evenly on your shoulders and both of your arms will be free to use the chairbacks for support.

48. Consider shipping heavy luggage or packages ahead (by UPS or an other shipping service) to your destination. Hotels will accept your packages prior to check-in. Contact your hotel to find out their procedures and to alert them of your plans.

At Your Destination

49. When you arrive at your hotel, gather pamphlets, local sightseeing maps, and other reading material about the area and retire to your room. Then spend some time relaxing and reading about the surroundings before heading out.

50. Extra blankets and pillows are available by calling the front desk of the hotel. Hotel personnel will deliver the items to your room.

51. If you forget personal items like a toothbrush, toothpaste, or shaver, ask the staff at the front desk whether they have these "complimentary" items for their guests.

52. Your hotel room "key" now looks like a credit card and contains your coded room information. However, if magnetic purse clasps, magnetic sunglass clips, or your cell phone come in contact with the card, they can clear the coded information and the card will no longer open your door. The front desk will be able to recode your card.

53. When you arrive at a sightseeing destination, ask for a map of the layout of the building or property and use the information to find the most accessible route to where you want to go, the handicapped restrooms, rest areas, and restaurant/food facilities.

Traveling by Car

54. To determine whether an exit off the highway will be to the right or to the left, watch the position of the small exit number panels on the top of road signs. If the small panel is on the right side of the sign, it's a right-lane exit ramp. If it's on the left side, it's a left-lane exit ramp.

55. Odd-numbered highways go north and south, whereas even-numbered roads go east and west.

56. When you travel, take along your personal state-issued disabled handicapped placard and hang it from your rearview mirror when you park the car. Disabled parking permits are honored in most states; you may use the placard on a rental car or in a car in which you are a passenger. If you forget to bring your permit with you, your only option may be to visit the nearest Department of Motor Vehicles office and request a temporary permit or contact the local police department to discuss your options. Don't be surprised if they may want to see a doctor's letter certifying your disability or medical condition.

57. If you need to travel with food or medication that must be refrigerated, take along a travel cooler that plugs into your vehicle's cigarette lighter. About the size of a mini refrigerator, it will keep medication, food, and drinks cool while you are driving and maintain that cool temperature without ice for several hours unplugged. Alternating current adaptors are available for home and hotel use. These are available in outdoor and discount department stores.

58. If you tend to get cold in the car while everyone else is comfortable, a Car Cozy Car Blanket plugs into your vehicle's cigarette lighter and provides extra warmth. A variety of sizes and styles are available at local stores.

59. If you travel by car with children, take along a jump rope, flying disc, balls, roller skates, or other toys they can use to work off excess energy when you stop at rest areas.

Traveling by Air

60. If you're traveling through an unfamiliar airline terminal and you're concerned about locating special services like companion/family

bathrooms, the First Aid station, food services, and rest areas for travelers with special needs, search the Internet for an up-to-date airport layout and pertinent information.

61. If you travel with a battery-operated mobility device, the airline will want to know what type of battery it uses. Carry documentation with you to avoid unnecessary delays and problems.

Airline Reservations

62. When making your airline reservations, a nonstop flight is preferable to one with connections, and a direct flight (two or more stops on one plane) is preferable to a connecting flight (two or more stops, two or more planes).

63. If you have connecting flights, make sure you have extra time between your connections to make the transfers easier and less stressful.

64. Many airlines let you confirm your seats online. If you are not sure what seating options are best for you, call the airline's toll-free number or ask the ticket agent about the options available on your plane.

65. Passengers needing assistance are often seated in the first row of the section, known as the *bulkhead seats*. These seats offer extra leg room. However, you must store your carry-on in the overhead compartment, not under your seat, and the seats do not have armrests that lift up.

Services Provided at the Airport

66. If it's available, check your luggage with an airline representative at the curb, instead of hauling it to the counter, or ask a porter to carry it for you.

67. Request a wheelchair at curbside check-in or at the inside ticket counter and eliminate standing in lines and walking long concourses. Conserve your energy for the day ahead.

68. When you use a (free) airport wheelchair, an airport employee will accompany you, help you navigate security, and locate needed services as well as accompany you directly to your gate.

Some porters accept tips for their service. Others don't. I always ask.

69. Planes no longer provide blankets and pillows, so be sure to take the creature comforts you may need.

70. Carry your prescription medications and other absolute necessities in your carry-on bag, so if your checked luggage is lost or misplaced or your medication gets spilled, you will still have what you need on hand.

71. With heightened airport security, passengers must present a driver's license, photo identification, or passport when checking in so that airport personnel can match you with the name on the ticket.

72. If you do not have a driver's license because you are unable to drive, call your state's Department of Motor Vehicle office to find out how to obtain a state picture identification card. If you don't have a copy of your (old or expired) driver's license, you will need a certified copy of your birth certificate or a passport and a copy of your signature on a document, such as a contract or tax return. Specific requirements differ from state to state, so call ahead.

73. If you have a disability, the Transportation Security Administration (TSA) offers personal screening by a Passenger Support Specialist (PSS). Contact TSA Cares at least 72 hours before you scheduled departure at 866-289-9673 or e-mail TSA-ContactCenter@TSA .dhs.gov. For more information check the TSA website (TSA.gov/travel/special-procedures).

Getting On (and Off) the Airplane

74. If you need to change your seat assignment, speak to your gate agent.

Because I am unable to walk, I need to be carried on the airplane in an aisle chair. If my assigned seat is toward the back of the plane, I ask the gate agent for a new seat assignment. With the attention to on-time departures, I explain that the further back I am in the plane, the longer it takes for me to get to my seat. My request is always honored and Dave and I are reseated.

75. If you are a slow walker, have balance problems, or other issues that make standing in line or boarding with other passengers difficult, discuss your needs with the gate agent and ask to pre-board. (You will be the first one on and the last one off.) If you arrive too late for preboarding, you will have to wait until everyone is on the plane before you board.

76. If you are traveling with your own three-wheeled scooter, wheelchair, or other mobility device, ask the gate agent to put a door-tag ticket on it so your device is delivered back to the jetway at your destination.

77. You may take your mobility device down the jetway to the door of the plane.

78. Once you're on the plane, someone from the baggage area will come up to the jetway and take your device down to the cargo hold.

79. If you have a manual-folding wheelchair, it can be stowed at your request in a closet in the cabin on any plane that has adequate storage; it has priority over any other baggage. Otherwise, it will be taken and put into the cargo hold of the plane.

80. If, like me, you are unable to transfer to an "aisle chair" (a narrow, straight-backed chair that fits between the aisles), your companion or airport personnel will lift and transfer you onto the chair. Airport personnel will carry you and the chair onto the plane. Once you are on the plane, the airport personnel will lift you out of the aisle chair and into your seat.

81. When you arrive at your destination, passengers needing assistance must wait until others are off the plane. Then you can leave the plane on the aisle chair; your scooter or wheelchair will be waiting for you in the jetway. Have your companion or airline personnel help you out of the aisle chair into your scooter and you're off!

On the Plane

82. If you think you might need to use the restroom while in-flight but would need a wheelchair to get there, you will need to use an onboard wheelchair. Because onboard wheelchairs are not used very often, be sure to let the flight crew know your needs before other passengers board with their carry-on luggage and fill the storage areas where the wheelchair may be stored.

83. Generally, airlines no longer serve meals to passengers. (Some may provide snack boxes for an additional fee.) Most still provide free snacks like pretzels, peanuts, packaged cookies, and candy bars. Be sure to take your own snacks like trail mix, power bars, dried fruits, and so on. If your plane is delayed for an extended time or you need to take medication with food, you'll be prepared.

84. If you're traveling on a long or international flight on which a meal will be served, be sure to contact the airline at least 48 hours in advance of your flight if you need a vegetarian, low-salt, kosher, or other special meal.

85. If you are one of the many people who experience pain or discomfort in their ears as a result of the changes in cabin pressure during takeoff and landing, try chewing gum or sipping a liquid through a straw. Swallowing helps to equalize the pressure inside your ears with that of the plane's cabin. You might want to speak to your physician to determine whether taking an over-the-counter antihistamine about half an hour before your flight time can prevent or lessen this discomfort.

Yes, it can be daunting to think about traveling and leaving all your creature comforts behind. However, I hope these tips and ideas provide a framework for planning a weekend getaway, a trip across the country, or around the world. You can do it! Just think of the memories and new adventures you'll have!

CHAPTER 15

Finding Help and Support

Today, modern multiple sclerosis therapies, not available when I was diagnosed, mean that people with MS are living longer, more productive lives. Some folks don't need or never will need devices or equipment to improve their ability to move, see, feel, hear, touch, or think. Even though treatments for my diagnosis, primary progressive multiple sclerosis (PPMS), are still very limited, many of us will, at some point, need items to help us accomplish everyday tasks.

In the early years of my diagnosis, my disability increased daily. I worried about the future: How would I manage my day-to-day activities and stay safe? It was depressing and disheartening. However, I became, and continue to be, tenacious about protecting some semblance of control in my life and using whatever resources, products, and services are available to me. And, in the process, I've learned that there is no end to the help that's available.

MS Organizations

1. The National Multiple Sclerosis Society (NMSS) provides a host of resources and connections to the latest research and treatments, peer-support groups, and online discussions, which will help you keep a positive attitude and give you hope for the future. They publish a quarterly magazine, *Momentum*, filled with encouraging first-person stories and informative articles by MS experts specifically about MS; past and present articles

are available online. Their website offers information on the latest research, helpful information for coping with MS symptoms, and has an "Ask an MS Navigator" through which you can ask questions of a network of people with MS as well as experts in the field.

A companion website (www.msconnection.org) connects you directly to discussion and support groups as well as professional and peer-to-peer counselors, and hosts an MS-related blog. An active message board forum is maintained at www.MSworld.org, which allows you to connect with others with MS who are facing similar challenges.

Local NMSS support groups and chapters nationwide offer educational programming and may have "loan closets" from which members may borrow devices to make daily living easier. To find out more about NMSS services in your area, contact them at 800-FIGHT MS (344-4867) or at www.NationalMS Society.org.

2. The Multiple Sclerosis Association of America (MSAA) provides many free services to make living with MS easier, including a helpline staffed by trained MS specialists; educational videos; a lending library that includes safety, mobility, and cooling equipment; and the My MS Manager app. MSAA publishes *The Motivator*, an MS-specific publication for coping with the challenges of MS and offers educational programs nationwide (800-532-7667; www .myMSAA.org).

3. The MS Foundation is dedicated to improving the quality of life for those affected by MS, including family and caregivers. Free services include a toll-free helpline staffed by case workers and peer counselors, educational programs, homecare services, support groups, assistive technology programs, publications, and a comprehensive website. All services are free to anyone affected by MS (800-225-6495; www.msfocus.org).

4. The Consortium of MS Centers is an organization for health care providers that facilitates and shares research in the field of MS (201-487-1050; www.MScare.org).

Online MS Communities

5. EverydayHealth.com/multiple-sclerosis is a blog contributed to by people with MS.

6. MSbloggers.com is a place where bloggers with MS can find each other.

7. MScando.org provides "whole person, whole health, whole community" programs and events encouraging people with MS, as well as their support and family members, to have a "can do" attitude for living well with MS.

8. ActiveMSers.org concentrates on info about staying active with MS by providing tips, product reviews, and social media interaction. The blog and forum provide encouragement and a place to find a listening ear when you feel overwhelmed.

9. Patientslikeme.com is a health data-sharing website that puts you in touch with others with chronic illness to enable you to share experiences and gain knowledge to better manage your condition. Search the site for "MS" and a variety of MS topics will appear.

National and Community-Based Support Services and Resources

10. Call the United Way 2-1-1 Information and Referral Line. Most U.S. communities can call 211 to connect to human service providers in your area. Consultants can turn your "where do I find help for . . . " questions into a list of agencies and resources where you will find answers for everything from basic human needs (food, clothing, shelter), to physical and mental health resources, and employment support.

11. Aging and Disability Resource Center (ADRC) counselors provide information and assistance regarding local agencies that offer services in health, employment, finances, transportation, as

well as in-home and long-term care options for those with chronic conditions like MS. Every county in the United States is served by an ADRC. Contact your state or county department of health and social services to be directed to the nearest ADRC office, or search online for ADRC + your state.

12. Disability.gov is a U.S. government website that provides extensive information on living independently with limitations. Their *Guide to Assistive and Accessible Technologies* provides evaluation methods and information on assistive and accessible technology that can make living and working with a disability easier. The site also offers quick links to state and financial loan programs to fund assistive devices.

13. The National Library Service for the Blind and Physically Handicapped sponsors "That all may read . . .," a free library program of Braille and audio materials distributed through a national network of cooperating libraries. If you (or someone you love) are unable to read, to hold a book, or turn a page as a result of physical limitations or a severe dysfunction that prevents you from reading in a normal manner, contact them to see whether you are eligible for this service (Library of Congress; 202-707-5100/800-424-8567; TTY 202-707-0744; www.loc.gov/nls).

14. The National Rehabilitation Information Center (NARIC) is the library for the National Institute on Disability, Independent Living, and Rehabilitation Research and a portal for finding information on a variety of topics. Their REHABDATA database includes over 80,000 documents covering physical, mental, and psychiatric disabilities; MS; independent living; vocational rehabilitation; assistive technology; disability law; employment; and social security to name a few (800-346-2742; TTY 301-459-5984; www.naric.com).

15. *The Complete Directory for People with Disabilities* is an exhaustive guide and resource for empowering people with disabilities to succeed at work, school, and in the community. The table of contents and sample pages are available online. To review the latest copy of the book, visit your local library or rehabilitation center

(published by Grey House Publishing; 800-562-2139; 518-789-8700; www.greyhouse.com/disabilities.htm).

16. The Disabilities Resource Community website is designed for people with disabilities, their family members, and caregivers. The website is a forum for these individuals to ask questions, share resources, and build community around the things that matter most (www.disabilityresource.org).

Locating Products to Keep You Independent

Today, many new (and some old) helpful products are readily available in stores. However, sometimes the products are so unique, they're difficult to find. Other times, you may not even be aware that such a product exists.

In each chapter, you'll find specific products pertinent to that chapter. However, there are many company websites that provide a variety of products covering many different categories. Because product offerings change from time to time and new products are added, search the companies listed here (and other sites you may find), to locate products and equipment to meet your needs. Search terms might include the following: "devices for accessible living," "accessibility aids & ideas," "aids to daily living," "independent living," or "aging in place." Be sure to compare prices, read product reviews, and look over the return policy.

www.Ableware.com
www.ActiveForever.com
www.AgingCare.com
www.AllegroMedical.com
www.BruceMedical.com
www.CaregiverProducts.com
www.EasierLiving.com
www.ElderDepot.com
www.ElderStore.com
www.healthcraftproducts.com
www.healthproductsforyou.com
www.healthykin.com

www.IndependentLiving.com
www.LifewithEase.com
www.LiveOakMed.com
www.Maddak.com
www.maxiaids.com
www.NCMedical.com
www.pattersonmedical.com
www.thewright-stuff.com

Selecting the Right Product

17. Consider getting an assessment of how well you handle the activities of daily living (dressing, grooming, eating, food preparation, exercising, and more). Ask your doctor for a referral to an occupational therapist (OT) who can provide this assessment and suggest products and services to help you accomplish difficult tasks more easily. If your needs vary from time to time or if your condition is progressing, some products may be better choices than others.

I know that every few years, I consult an OT to help me stay as independent as I can. Sometimes the therapist makes a home visit to see me in my own environment. Ask your doctor to refer you to an OT to advise you regarding aids that meet your needs, now and long term.

18. Whenever products are recommended, it's vitally important that you consider and evaluate the product before you purchase it. You should choose what YOU feel is best for you, your lifestyle, and your budget.

When it was (highly) recommended that I get a power "tilt in space," wheelchair (upward of $35,000), I had three different chairs delivered to my home, each for a 10-day trial period. The company even sent representatives to show me how to use the complicated, computerized controls. In the end, I decided that these power wheelchairs were too big and too complicated for me to handle. In fact, they actually decreased my independence. Instead, I opted for a $3,500, three-wheeled Amigo®

scooter with a modified seating system. As guilty as I felt for "wasting the salesmen's time," I'm immensely happy that I followed my instincts and chose the product that was best for me.

Try Before You Buy

The example of my wheelchair experience shows that it's costly to purchase products and special equipment. You want to avoid making a mistake, so I recommend you try before you buy. Over the years, I've found numerous ways to try products before I buy them.

19. Contact your local independent living center (ILC). Every community in the United States is part of a national network of community-based, nonprofit, ILCs that serve people of all ages and disabilities and their families. Most centers have adaptive gadgets and devices that you may borrow and try for a while at no cost, and a vast computer database of the companies and manufacturers that make these products.

Your local library, hospital, or social services agency should be able to assist you in finding the nearest ILC. For a national directory of Independent Living Centers, contact the National Council on Independent Living (202-207-0334; www.ncil.org).

20. Your state or county may maintain a listing of organizations with loan closets and medical equipment and healthcare product recycling programs or provide links to agencies that temporarily lend or donate equipment and supplies to people in need. Contact your local health and social services agency or ADRC for a list of resources near you. To locate the ADRC in your area search "ADRC" + your state.

21. Many national organizations (often related to your diseases), medical condition, or disability), senior centers, and social service agencies have loan closets, lending libraries, or health equipment loan programs (HELP) that let you borrow products (short term.) Generally, the items are free to borrow, however, large items like wheelchairs might incur a rental cost or "donation."

22. Hospitals and rehabilitation centers have Occupational Therapy departments that are supplied with equipment and products for patients to use as they recover from their medical issues. Seeing a hospital OT will give you access to their products.

23. Check out home health stores in the community. Often they're affiliated with your clinic or health maintenance organization (HMO), and will work with your healthcare team and insurance companies to see whether the equipment is covered by your insurance. Some stores have large showrooms with equipment on display for you to try. If an item you are looking for is not on display, ask whether the equipment can be ordered for trial.

24. Home-improvement stores, especially those that have showrooms, may have adapted tub and shower combinations, closet adaptations, grab bars, decorative paddle-handled faucets, and more. When purchasing appliances or other big-ticket items, try out different products to be certain you can reach the controls and have the strength and dexterity to operate the switches, open doors, press buttons, and so on.

25. Consider asking your friends and neighbors whether they have a specific item you'd like to try; maybe they'll let you borrow it.

When I was in bed for 3½ months with an early-stage bedsore, my neighbor let me borrow her bed table and a special book holder.

26. If you belong to a homeowner's association (HOA) that has a newsletter, consider asking whether someone has the item you are interested in seeing, trying out, or borrowing.

27. Look on Craig's list.

When I was no longer able to use my standing frame (a device that helps you stand up), I posted it on the website and sold it to someone who could use it.

28. Check out Pinterest.com to find thousands of photos and ideas to inspire you. Maybe you'll create the product you need!

Purchasing Durable Medical Equipment

29. With a doctor's prescription, durable medical equipment (DME) is typically covered by your healthcare insurance. Walkers, crutches, wheelchairs, power scooters, seat lifts, hospital beds, home oxygen equipment, and so on are considered as DME.

30. Insurance companies have limits on how often they will purchase some equipment (walker, wheelchair, or scooter) for you. You want to be absolutely certain that you consider your personal comfort using the device, as well as the size, weight, portability and transportability, ease of operating the controls/switches, and whether or not you plan to use the product indoors or out.

31. Some people find operating a battery-powered mobility device intimidating and scary. Speaking from 30+ years of personal experience, power-operated vehicles are not nearly as easy to maneuver as they look. People whose reaction time is diminished and/or whose mental processing is slower than "normal," may find that power wheelchairs and scooters may not be the best choice.

32. If others need to manage a manual wheelchair, make certain the handles are in a comfortable position for pushing and that the chair is light enough to get it into and out of the car without causing an injury.

33. A transport chair, which has four wheels of the same size, may be an appropriate choice for someone who needs a wheelchair, but is unable to propel a manual wheelchair. Transport chairs are less expensive than a manual wheelchair, are portable, lightweight, and designed for short-term use.

Index

About the Author

SHELLEY PETERMAN SCHWARZ and her husband, Dave, live in Madison, Wisconsin. They've been married since 1969 and enjoy being the parents of two adult children, Jamie and Andrew. They have five grandchildren.

At the time of her multiple sclerosis diagnosis in 1979, Shelley was working part time as a teacher of the deaf. Two years later, because of the effects of progressive MS, she retired. In 1985, when a story she wrote appeared in *Inside MS*, the magazine of the National Multiple Sclerosis Society, a new career was born. Since then, Shelley has published nearly 1,000 articles and received numerous awards, including the Mother of the Year from the Wisconsin chapter of the National MS Society and the Spirit of the American Woman Award from JC Penney, and she was named a Woman of Distinction by the YWCA.

Shelley's nationally syndicated column, "Making Life Easier," and features have appeared in newspapers, magazines, books, and international publications, including *Momentum* (National Multiple Sclerosis Society), *The Motivator* (Multiple Sclerosis Association of America), *MS Focus* (MS Foundation), *MS Canada*, *MS Life* (Australia), *Family Circle*, *Arthritis Today* (Arthritis Foundation), *Neurology Now* (American Academy of Neurology), *Friendly Wheels* (Amigo Mobility International) and more. Her tips are available on numerous websites as well.

In 1997, the National Arthritis Foundation, Inc., commissioned Shelley to write *250 Tips for Making Life with Arthritis Easier* based on her "Making Life Easier" column. *More Making Life Easier* books followed:

Dressing Tips and Clothing Resources for Making Life Easier (Attainment Company, 2000)
Multiple Sclerosis: 300 Tips for Making Life Easier (Demos Medical Publishing, 1999, 2006)
Parkinson's Disease: 300 Tips for Making Life Easier (Demos Medical Publishing, 2002, 2006)
Organizing Your IEPs (Individualized Educational Plan for Special Education Students; Attainment Company, 2005)
Memory: Tips for Making Life Easier (Attainment Company, 2005)

Shelleys' words and stories also appear in the following books:

Parenting: When the Parent Has a Disability (Cheever Publishing, 1989)
A Second Chicken Soup for the Woman's Soul (Health Communications, Inc., 1998)
Jewish Mothers Tell Their Stories: Acts of Love and Courage (The Haworth Press, Inc., 2000)
Amazingly Simple Lessons We Learned After 50 (M. Evans and Co., Inc., 2001)
Mental Sharpening Stones: Cognitive Challenges with MS (Demos Health, 2009)
Primary Progressive Multiple Sclerosis: What You Need to Know (DiaMedica, 2010)
Child Development, 14th ed. (McGraw-Hill Education, 2013)

In 1995, Shelley self-published a book titled, *Blooming Where You're Planted: Stories from the Heart*. The previously published essays chronicle her journey of change and self-discovery following her MS diagnosis. A professional speaker, Shelley's philosophy of life is to find solutions to whatever problems she faces and to help others do the same. Her motivational and inspirational keynotes help audiences see challenges in their lives as opportunities for personal growth. She shares her message of hope and teaches audiences how to "bloom wherever they're planted."

Visit www.MakingLifeEasier.com to read more of Shelley's tips and stories. Her e-mail address is: Shelley@MakingLifeEasier.com